Cancer

It's a Good Thing I Got It!

ALWAYS REMEMBER
THAT TODAY IS SOMEDAY!

DAVID A. KOOP

Cancer

It's a Good Thing I Got It!

The Life Story of a Very Lucky Man

David A. Koop

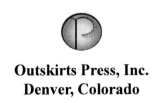

Outskirts Press, Inc.
Denver, Colorado

Outskirts Press, Inc.
http://www.outskirtspress.com

Paperback ISBN: 978-1-4327-7448-6
Hardback ISBN: 978-1-4327-7578-0

Outskirts Press and the "OP" logo are trademarks belonging to Outskirts Press, Inc.

PRINTED IN THE UNITED STATES OF AMERICA

Dedication

They say that God never gives us more than we can handle.

That may be true . . . but I'm here to tell you that if it is true, it does not stop him from redefining what you can handle and pushing right up to that new limit.

One thing I know is, unless you have lived through it . . . you just have no idea and there are no words I can write to help you truly understand. So let's just go with it was a horrible slog.

I also know that I owe my life to my son, Christopher. He is the reason I am alive . . . PERIOD! My son was only six when I got my news. I told every doctor who would listen and even the ones who did not believe me, that I had waited 41 years for my son to come along and I was not going to leave him now. I would do everything they asked . . . chemo, radiation, surgery and a wheelchair if need be, anything and everything . . . except die! I had waited too long to run off and leave my son now.

So I told the doctors, "I will get used to the idea of fighting cancer . . . You guys get used to the idea that I'm not going anywhere." As you start this journey you meet other people on a similar journey. As I spoke with them and looked into their eyes, I could see those who had given up and those who had a reason to live. Everyone with empty eyes . . . is gone.

This book talks about my life and my slog with cancer, but it's also about living life and the rewards I got for hanging in there. Not just the time to raise my son, but also my wife, Carrie. She has won her own battle with cancer and now we are going through life side-by-side; she and her sons Mitchel and Garret, and Christopher and I accepting the challenges and relishing in the adventures. Living life to the fullest every single day.

Life is precious, don't ever look back and say I wish I would have done this or I wish I had done that. Do it now. Tell the people in your life that you love them, right now. Treat every day as if it were your last, because you just never know!

We've all heard people say, "Someday I'm going to do this or someday I'm going to do that." You've probably even said it yourself. But we really, really have no idea when our time is up. So what I say to you is… ***Today is Someday!***

Today, once again, just like every day, I am telling Christopher, Garret, Mitchel and Carrie that I love them all. I'm dedicating this book to them because Christopher kept me alive then, and they are all my reasons for living now.

Table of Contents

Prologue

A wise man should consider that health is the greatest of human blessings, and learn how by his own thought to derive benefit from his illnesses.

~ Hippocrates

Blame It On The Ostriches

It was just a normal day, no different than any other. There was no way to know that the events of that evening would change my life forever.

As I got dressed to go out for the evening, I decided to wear my ostrich skin cowboy boots. You know how employers always have some way to reward and motivate their employees, such as lottery tickets, bonuses, trips, or even a new car? Well, when you are the boss, there is no one to reward you. So I learned to set specific goals with specific rewards to help keep me motivated. The ostriches were one such reward, and I had not worn them in quite a while.

After I finished getting dressed, I swung by and picked up the lady that I was dating at the time. We were on our way to a wine event at the State Fairgrounds in Salem, Oregon. I owned several different businesses at the time, one of which was a vineyard supply company, so I knew many of the people there. I was also looking for new wines to add to the online wine, gift baskets and Oregon food products website that I had recently started.

It was a fun event, seeing old friends and making new ones, tasting wines and good food and listening to live music. We walked up and down the aisles, seeing new label art and tasting those wines and catching up with old friends and acquaintances.

About halfway through the evening my back began to hurt. It felt like severe sciatic nerve pain. It wasn't the first time I had that problem in my life, but this time it came on fast and hard. It was like a Samurai warrior had violently inserted his sword into me, thrusting it up my spine on the inside of me. I had never felt such pain. It was agonizing.

Within a few minutes, this big tough man (6'3" and 300 pounds) was standing in the middle of the Jackman Long building with tears running down my face, unable to move.

Since we had been dating for several months, my date knew that I had problems with back pain on occasion, but she had never seen me like this, no one had, not even me. She felt completely helpless, you know how it is when someone you care about is hurting and there is nothing that you can do. She gave me physical support by holding my arm and giving me herself to lean on. She also tried with her words to provide as much comfort as she could. Unfortunately there were no words or physical support that was going to make the pain go away. With the help of my date and a kind stranger, we headed out to my truck.

Each and every step I took caused that sword to be rammed ever harder. An excruciating pain would take my breath away with each shuffle of my feet. It wasn't a long walk back to the truck; luckily it was parked just across the street, as close to the exit door as possible, but it still took me over 30 minutes to make it. My date drove us back to my house and installed me in bed.

I have dealt with pain most of my adult life. Due to skiing accidents, poor decisions in my youth (you really should use proper body mechanics when lifting), and a degenerative disc disease, lower back pain was nothing new. This pain, though, was extreme.

Normally when my back acted up, it meant that I would be bedridden for anywhere from one to three days taking pain pills, using the heating pad, soaking in the hot tub and getting better. Mentally, that's what I was ready for. But, come Monday, I was no better. In fact, the pain was a little worse. So I called my doctor, and he got me in straightaway.

On February 14, 2006, I explained to my doctor what I had been going through. I shared with him that I had not worn my ostrich skin cowboy boots for an awfully long time. I thought maybe the new position of my back with the heel of the boots walking on the concrete floors for several hours was the cause of this problem. He wasn't sure if that was the cause, but he could tell there was something seriously wrong, so he scheduled me for an MRI. On February 23rd, I was at the Salem Radiology Clinic.

I'd had several MRIs in my life, and from the progress of this one it was obvious to me that there was something seriously wrong. A couple of things caused me to be concerned. First after the technician completed the MRI he said, "I need to call your doctor," then came back and said, "We need to do this study again." After the new MRI he said. "We are going to need to do this yet again but this time with a contrast dye." For the contrast MRI they inject a radioactive dye into your blood stream to give the doctors an entirely different view. The dye they were using this time is absorbed more by tumors, they call it "take up" and it causes the tumors to light up on the films as "hot spots."

Even though I knew there was a problem, I was not sure what the problem was since the technicians don't tell you what they see. You have to wait for the radiologist to read the results and then meet with your primary care physician to get the news. I just assumed that my disc problems had finally gotten so bad that it was time for surgery on my herniated discs. Meanwhile, life went on.

I had a trade show coming up for the wine business, but with my level of pain it was impossible to work that show by myself. I asked my best friend, Tito, to come up from Oxnard, California to help me work the trade show. Luckily the show was in Eugene, Oregon, only about an hour south of where I live in Salem.

Tito was happy to fly up and help, and it's a good thing he did, because I spent three quarters of the time up in the hotel suite lying on the bed suffering intense pain. The following Monday after the show, Tito took me to the doctor's office to get the results of the MRI. Tito does not much care for doctors and medicine so he waited in the car. When I came out I guess he could tell by my expression or the lack of color in my face that something was not right. He asked me what the doctor had said, but I could not reply. "What did he say, David?" he asked again.

His question took me back into the office where I had been just minutes ago with my primary care physician, Dr. Michael Kelber. Dr. Kelber has been my doctor since December of 2005, when I had moved to him because of the substandard care I had been receiving for my previous doctor. Lucky for me, my neighbor was head of medical staff services at our local hospital. We talked regularly about things, as close neighbors do, and things happening in my life from a medical standpoint came up on occasion. She would ask did they do this. Did they do that test? Are they treating you for X or Y? The answer was always, "No."

Finally, after lots of prodding, I changed doctors and I was very happy with the change; I know that the quality of my life was drastically improved long term by the change. My new doctor and I hit it off right away and I felt completely comfortable with the care that I received from him. He has a no-nonsense approach, very straight-forward, clear and direct, just the way I like it.

I turned to my friend, looked in his eyes, and as I burst into tears I told him, "He said -- I'm going to die."

"Bullshit," Tito said. "He didn't tell you were going to die. What did he say?" Through the tears I tried to explain to him what the doctor had explained to me. When Dr. Kelber came into the room he did not have that smile that he normally wore. He avoided eye contact and pulled a chair up close to mine. He had a sorrowful look on his face and he said, "I wish I had better news; it's bad . . . it's really bad." He said that I had a tumor at the base of my spine about the size of a small peach. There was not going to be a good outcome and that I needed to get my affairs in order. He wished that he had better news and wished he could tell me anything else, but this was bad, this was really, really bad.

But, there was some good news at least…The good news? You know there is always good news! Well, the good news was that we couldn't really blame it on the ostriches after all.

Growing Up

Chapter 1

This life is yours. Take the power to choose what you want to do and do it well. Take the power to love what you want in life and love it honestly. Take the power to walk in the forest and be a part of nature. Take the power to control your own life. No one else can do it for you. Take the power to make your life happy.

~ Susan Polis Schutz

My Mom

As the words of my doctor echoed in my mind I started to think about my life. What if it really was over? What would happen to my son Christopher? He was only six years old. I hadn't gotten anywhere near enough time to raise him. It made me think of my first memories as a child.

The very first memory I have is all three of my older sisters and me sitting on a hard wood bench in some really big, old building. Each of my sisters had been taken away down the hall, one by one. It is my turn now, and an older lady takes me by the hand and leads me away from the bench. As I looked back over my shoulder I saw my three sisters sitting on that well-worn bench.

I was led into a room that seemed to this little boy of only five years old to be huge. There was an older man sitting behind the desk. I was placed on an oversized chair across the desk from him. He asked me questions, most of which I don't remember. But there was one question that I do remember, the same question that this same man had asked my three older sisters.

This was my introduction to the legal system. The well-worn bench was in the hall of the Fresno County Courthouse and the old man behind the desk was a judge. The question that judge asked of all four of us was, "Do you want to live with your mom or your dad?" I gave the same answer that my sisters said that they gave, that we wanted to live with our mother.

At five years old I was far too young to understand everything that was going on, but I do know the result. Custody was given to my Dad. I have never asked why my dad got custody; as I got older it was never that important. It's not like knowing was going to magically snap us back in time and make it turn out differently. There was also the chance that dredging it up would bring pain to people that I love and care about.

I have no recollection of day-to-day life as a young child, but I do know that my mother was lost to me. Prior to this judicial interference we were with our mother when she finally had to throw in the towel on her marriage to my Dad. I recall a little, bits and pieces. A few other small memories I gained from my sisters and even a little from my Mom. The time we spent, about a year, living at grandma's Belmont Road house on the west side of Fresno, a pool, horses, Mom and my three sisters. Then Mom got us our own house on Buckingham Road (still in Fresno) where we lived until we were given to our Dad.

Mom says I can ask her anything, and she means it, but I can see when I am with her or hear the pain on the phone when I call, I just don't want to take her there. We have talked about those lost years more during the writing of this book than ever before, but I think you will understand that I love my mother and I don't wish to cause her pain. Like me, due to her own failing health she is forced to try to live each day with pain, physical pain, from moderate to severe. So I choose not to add heaping helpings of emotional pain on top of that. It does not matter, that was then and this is now. I love her and she loves me!

I was five years old that Christmas night when my Dad, custody order in hand, came to Grandma's house and took us away from my mother. I only have two memories as a child of my mother after that. The first was coming home from school one day and seeing an MG in the driveway. A very cool sports car and it was a convertible. It turned out that it belonged to my mother. I can't remember how long she stayed; I just remember the car in the driveway.

The second memory I have is of my mother and her new husband picking up my three sisters and me at my Dad's house in a much bigger car. They took us on a vacation to Santa Cruz. As best as I can remember we had a good time. I am not sure how old I was but I think I was around 11 or 12 years old. There was one small problem at the beach where my sister thought she was in big trouble. The four of us were at the beach and I was riding a skim board, a round thin board that you throw on the beach as the wave is moving out.

Not being very good at this sport I took more than a few falls. When my sister Bonnie saw my knee she freaked. It was massively swollen and badly bruised, so back to the house we went. My knee works fine so I guess it got better, and I don't remember what we did for treatment, but from the time of that vacation on I don't remember spending any other time with my Mom.

Fast-forward to 1984 and you find me at the ripe old age of 25 living in Denver, Colorado. I was working hard to develop and build National Legal Shield. NLS was a prepaid legal plan company. Prepaid legal plans are similar to dental or medical insurance, in that you pay a premium and receive specified benefits. There are many different kinds of plans out there; the pure insurance models as well as affinity discount plans, with hybrids in-between. With NLS you could get a plan for yourself as an individual or family, a business plan for commercial needs and employee benefit plans, provided to the employees by their employer. All of NLS's plans allowed people to get quality legal services at a cost that they could afford.

For reasons I can't explain, I started thinking about my Mom. I had not seen or heard from her for years and years. I decided that I wanted to find her, to reconnect. I made some phone calls and got my mom's number.

It was a Sunday afternoon when I dialed the number for my Mom. She answered and a two-hour conversation followed. This was a great first step at reconnecting with my mother. We talked about anything and everything, and nothing was out of bounds. From "How is your sex life?" to "Who do you favor in the upcoming election?" I am happy to report that we agree in our thoughts about sex, as we are both in favor of an active sex life with a loving partner. But when it comes to politics we get in spirited discussions due to the fact that we are on opposite sides of most issues. This always provides an opportunity to debate the issues of the day. Every Sunday after that, Mom and I talked on the phone. It was a hole in my life that was slowly filling up each and every Sunday.

We were developing marketing offices for National Legal Shield during the time my Mom and I reconnected. NLS was bringing in people from around the country who wanted to learn how to develop a business in the prepaid legal industry. In the winter of 1984 I asked Mom if she would like to join our next training class in Denver. It would give her an opportunity to see what her son did for a living.

So during the spring of 1985, my Mom flew into Denver as one of several members of the current training group. We had decided to keep her identity secret until completion of the training class. She was involved in each and every activity day and night for a full week of training, including those ever-popular role-playing sessions. It was not all work, though. Mom and her classmates got to eat the official "second best" cheeseburger in Colorado as well as enjoying prime seats while watching the Denver Gold play to a win in an Arena Football League game. After the Graduation ceremony we revealed to everyone that she was my mother and that we were reconnecting after years of separation. Everyone was very emotional and wished us well as we ventured on in our lives, together once again.

Once the class was over the others flew home, but Mom stayed and we spent the next week getting to know each other on a more personal level. We traveled to several areas of interest in Colorado, such as Red Rocks Amphitheater and the cool city of Morrison, where I got a necklace for my Mom; it had a miniature pinecone dipped in gold as a pendant. It's a gift she still cherishes today as a reminder of our time spent reconnecting.

I learned so many things about my mother and her life, enough to fill another book. But here are a few highlights; my Mom was recognized, along with her partner, as Humboldt County's Person of the Year for their work with the homeless. One of the first people to provide marijuana brownies to AIDS patients in San Francisco . . . that's right my Mom! She also liked to hang with celebrities for a good cause, like the time she was arrested alongside Bonnie Raitt as they marched to protect the old growth forests. Now in 2011, people are making a big fuss about Sarah Palin and her commercial fishing . . . But my Mom was a commercial fisherman long before Sarah even thought about politics, let alone fishing.

Somebody once asked me, why did you wait so long to reach out to her? I don't really know for sure, I can only speculate. I was a very aggressive Type A personality, chasing my dreams, building my fortune. She had not been there, not by her choice, just the way it worked out. I did not think about it, until that Sunday, and yes I wish I had done it much sooner.

Mom still lives on the northern California coast, where we visit her regularly. We continue to talk on the phone and yes, nothing is off limits in our conversations.

Chapter 2

Sometimes you've got to let everything go – purge yourself. If you are unhappy with anything… whatever is bringing you down, get rid of it. Because you'll find that when you're free, your true creativity, your true self comes out.

~ Tina Turner

My Dad

It was long before iPods, no ear buds for me. I had those giant old time headphones on with the volume turned way up. I was listening to Cat Stevens on my cassette player. I liked the whole tape but I was playing one song over and over again; Father and Son. The words of that song spoke to me so clearly. They echoed the very problem that I had been having with my father. "How can I try to explain? When I do he turns away again, it's always been the same old story. From the moment I could talk I was ordered to listen. I know I have to go away."

I would sit in my room, headphones on, volume up, and listen to that song over and over and over yet again. Repeatedly asking myself why did it have to be that way? My Dad had raised me to be an active, intelligent and engaged person. A person who had thoughts, ideas and questions; all of which I wanted, no, needed, to share. It was not a feeling that I chose. It was a natural part of my being. Those needs still exist in me to this day.

I have tried hard to understand my Dad and the things that happened between us, and the things that still do not exist between us. I do not have a relationship with my Dad. It's not because I don't want one and it's not because I have not tried. It's not something that my Dad wants. It's like they say, "It takes two to Tango!" Speaking of the Tango, looking back, I don't think I've ever seen my Dad dance. I am trying right now but I can't remember him ever laughing either, how very sad.

When people ask me how I am able to be such a good dad to Christopher I half jokingly say, "Easy, I ask myself, what would my Dad do? Then I do the opposite." I did learn some valuable lessons from my father though. Here are a few of them. If you took it out, when you're done put it back. If you unlocked it, when you're done, re-lock it. If you borrow something return it in as good a condition or better than when you got it. Be on time. (He would tell me over and over. You can show up to work every day an hour early, year after year. But if you show up five minutes late one day, you are still late. Take care of your tools and your tools will take care of you.

These were all important things to learn; the common-sense things of life that so many of the young employees applying at my companies seem never to have been taught in their life. But, I wanted more than just these common sense lessons from my dad.

What I wanted and needed was an emotional relationship. By most measurements I have been a success in life. When I was young I did well in school. I was active in after school activities, football, track and band. My Dad never came to any of these. In business I have had major successes, even appearing on ABC's Good Morning America. Never once have I heard my Dad say, "Good job" or "I am proud of you." Obviously I succeeded without it, but my soul yearned for that recognition from my father . . . It has never come.

I have spent a lifetime asking myself why. Why won't he talk with me? Why won't he come see me? Yes, I travel to see him on occasion and he will spend an hour chatting about nothing of any true meaning, usually the weather or something just as unimportant.

When my mother and I reconnected she shared the story of her and my Dad breaking up. In that story she told me about how my Dad had ceased to exist after a medical procedure he was put through after an accident. My Mom said that after the electroshock therapy, my Dad, as she had known him, was gone. His personality disappeared. It was like the loving, caring man that she had met and married died that day.

So I tell myself that the reason my Dad won't share his emotions with me is because he can't. Sometimes that works to ease the pain in my heart. Most of the time I can't help but think about my simple two-part credo for success, "Decide, then Do." Why doesn't he just pick up the phone and call me? Why doesn't he just shoot me a quick email? Old school, that's right, he is old school! OK, then why not pick up a pen and a pad of paper and write a letter, or even just a note. Is a birthday card too much to ask?

I can hear your questions. What about you, David? Are you doing the things you need to in order to have a relationship with your dad? To answer you, yes I am. Yes I have . . . and to the day my dad or I die, yes I will. The last big step I took involved this book. After writing the chapter "Sometimes You Really Do Get What You Wish For," I thought, I want to share this great memory with my Dad and let him know just how much it meant to me as a kid. I wanted him to know that it still moved my heart as a grown man. So I drove to central California and gave my Dad a copy of that chapter. He did not say thank you . . . not a big surprise. That was several months ago, and I have still not heard a single word. Not a "Thank you," not "Wow I had no idea that meant so much to you," or even, "You know that is one of my fond memories too." Nothing…it hurts.

My earliest memories with my dad start about the same time as they did with my mom, in the courthouse. After the court reached its decision, my sisters and I ended up living with my dad and new stepmom a in a small white farmhouse on the east side of the Easton, a small town about 25 minutes south of Fresno.

There were a lot of people for such a small house. Three older sisters, three younger brothers, a stepmother, my dad and me, all sharing that house. My three older sisters; Jody, Bonnie, Susan and I shared the same parents. Brothers Jeff and Jamie were Janene's kids, my new stepmother. And our youngest brother Tommy was the loving result of Dad and Janene's new marriage. I have never referred to any of my siblings as "step this" or "half that." It's always been my brothers and my sisters. Some people have felt compelled to argue with me about this in the past but I figure since it's my life, how I think about it is the only thing that really matters. I have three older sisters and three younger brothers, and it will be that way forever.

I only remember one thing that happened at that little white house. It was small but it was surrounded by lots of farmland for us to play on and one day my brother Jeff decided he was going to push a red button. You see my dad liked to build dune buggies that we would take over to Pismo Beach on the California coast and race around the sand dunes. My Dad had put an automatic starter on the dune buggy. One day, Jeff, who was still in diapers, climbed up on the dune buggy and pushed the red button. The dune buggy was in gear and off it went. Not far across the field Jeff fell out of the dune buggy and it ran right over his head. Lucky for him the field of been freshly plowed. It removed a little bit of his hair, but mostly just pushed his head down into the freshly plowed earth. It scared everybody except Jeff. I don't think he liked the haircut, but he laughed about the ride!

Next we moved to a house on Clara Street on the west side of Easton, just a couple blocks up from the high school football stadium. I have a few more memories of life at this house, because that's mostly where I grew up. I remember one Christmas morning looking out the sliding glass doors into the backyard and seeing a pony tied up to the tree.

His name was Simon. My dad had rented the barn and 10 acres of pasture across the street. Our job that Christmas morning was to get Simon from our backyard, across the street through the barn and into the pasture. It seemed like a simple task. We didn't yet have the necessary tack to do it correctly, but my sister Sue took the rope and wrapped it around Simon's neck and his nose and made a handheld halter. It seemed like a pretty good system and Simon was very compliant. Somehow or another I was chosen to ride, so I was hoisted up onto the bare back of Simon as Sue led him out our gate, down the driveway and headed across the street to get to the pasture.

As we got to the middle of the street Simon decided that it was rodeo time and he started bucking. The first time he reared his head up it ripped that handheld halter right out of Sue's hand and all that was left was a young boy with no riding experience on the back of that pony. No saddle, no bridle and no halter, nothing but a handful of mane. On his second buck I was launched up into the air and landed flat on my back in the middle of the pavement. One heck of an introduction to our new pony on Christmas Day.

Another thing we quickly learned about Simon was he was a very polite pony. As you were galloping across the pasture if he would come to a small ditch, he would stop and let you go over first.

It was a lesson that we all had to learn on our own.

Simon soon got a new friend. His name was Daniel, a great big paint, and he was as far to the gentle side as Simon was to the wild side. It was safe for anyone, with or without experience to ride Daniel. If you even started to fall off he would stop to make sure you could right yourself in the saddle. And he was game for any kind of tricks. My soon to be brother-in-law Dan (Jody's boyfriend) could do the Indian pickup; he could run and jump on from behind. Daniel was just as patient as could be.

Just as the dune buggies had given way to the horses, horses soon gave way to sailboats. When my dad was younger, before he'd even gotten married, he had built a sailboat by hand. It was very well built and about 15' long if I remember correctly. I believe my dad did take it out for a sail or two before I was born but that sailboat lived for most of my life in a sand-filled swimming pool in the back of my grandparent's house. All of the grandkids would captain a voyage whenever they came over. More importantly, my grandparents no longer had to worry about any of the grandkids drowning in that pool. No one ever did that I know of but they did have enough fear to fill it up with sand.

All of our vacations, most of our weekends, and even some mid-week evenings were spent sailing. There were sailboat races. There were out of town regattas and there were my parent's friends with their families in tow, driving in a convoy to launch their boats for family vacations at the coast and faraway lakes. One of Janene's phrase's that I remember most is a classic, "You're going to have fun whether you like it or not!" Of the older kids in our house, I liked sailing the most and took to racing sailboats, as I grew older. None of the issues at home ever bothered me when I was out on the water in my own boat.

There's a saying I learned that "It's amazing how much smarter your parents get as you grow older." And I know that most, if not all, kids have trouble with their parents when they are growing up. But my dad and stepmom were not easy to live with. I believe in my heart that they tried the best that they knew how. When Janene and her two boys came into the family, Janene was just a handful of years older than my sister Jody. But yet she was supposed to be prepared to be in charge of a family of nine. In retrospect it seems like she might've been set up for failure. Ya think? My dad tried to raise me the way he was raised; children were to be seen and not heard. And if you got out of line you got the belt or the brush or whatever was handy.

He did not always need a tool to express his displeasure. The biggest impact on our family and me came from his behavior at the dinner table. If I was not eating the lima beans on my plate (or any other food item) my Dad would come up behind me and hit me in the head, hard enough to knock me sideways in my chair.

When this would start one or more of my sisters would jump up from the table screaming for him to stop as they ran out of the house to hide. They would do this in hopes of distracting Dad from me. They had lots of places to hide when they ran but Sue told me later that her favorite spot was the pigeon coop. She preferred the gentle cooing of the pigeons in stark contrast to the screaming and yelling and hitting going on at the dining table.

I admit it. One time, I asked for it. I was sick and tired of hearing about the "starving children in China" whenever I would not eat my lima beans or salmon patties. On one very memorable occasion I was ready for my stepmom. She started in on her starving children in China routine, and I reached into my pocket and slapped a $5 dollar bill down on the table and said, "Then ship it to them"… WHACK!! Oh but it was worth it!

I explained to Carrie when we got together that I was unable to fight with the kids about food at the dinner table. If someone did not like lima beans so be it. But it is just too painful for me to relive that part of my childhood. Lima beans… seriously, who really cares?

My sisters had their own troubles, and one by one they left the house before their 18th birthdays because of those troubles. I swore that I wasn't going to leave until I was 18, but things just didn't work out the way I had planned.

I was fifteen the first time I ran away, moving into an apartment in Fresno. I was sharing it with my girlfriend's best friend's boyfriend. (Wow that sounds like the beginning of a Jerry Springer episode-- but it wasn't.) I was going to high school during the day and doing janitorial work at night to pay my share of the rent. Finances were tight and I didn't even own a car. Not that it mattered since I didn't have a driver license either. So I rode my bike.

It was such a ridiculous sight, me pedaling my Peugeot eighteen-speed bike down the road in the middle of the night, with a vacuum cleaner, a bucket, mop and a rake hanging off the frame. As you imagine the sight, in your mind add the music track from the Wizard of Oz, the scene as the evil witch is riding her bike with Toto in the basket. You know . . . "Dunt, tadunt tada daa, dunt tadunt tada daa…" That's the music that was playing in my head as I rode through the night from job to job thinking how crazy the whole thing seemed.

I even got "pulled over" by the police on more than one occasion. At that time kids in Fresno less than 18 years of age were not supposed to be out alone after 10:00 pm, and here I was at 2:00 in the morning. It turned out that my verbal skills had developed early enough to keep me out of jail. In dealing with the police I learned early on if you had a good story you could get further, those stories filled with laughter kept me out of several police cars, except one day when my roommate got arrested.

I learned that part about the law, where if you are with someone who is committing or has committed a crime, you go for a ride downtown too. Seems my roommate's car had been seen at a burglary, and the police got his plate number. When they came to the apartment to arrest him, they found stolen items in his room. They also found a minor child (that was me!). So off to juvenile hall I went, as he was taken to jail.

It was an educational experience for me. First, the officer who was given the job of transporting me to juvenile hall was tired. He had me handcuffed with my hands behind my back. He grabbed the cuffs and lifted up until I was high on my tip toes and he explained that he was so tired that he would not chase after me. No, he was too tired to chase after me so if I ran he would just shoot me. He asked if I understood. Yes, I did, and no, I did not run, never even thought about it.

Next came my new "friends" in jail--a unique group of people that I was not used to being around. All the horrible things that you hear about that happen to the new kids in lockup flooded my mind. So when a rather large and well tattooed one asked what I was in for, I took my time and answered in the best delivery possible, "Murder . . . yeah . . . I killed my Dad. Not sure why they're locking me up though, he deserved it, you know." I figured if I was going to be spending nights with these folks I wanted them to think twice about bothering me.

At some point in the day the guard came in and said you have a visitor. When I got to the private visitors room I saw that it was my dad. He was angry, and never even bothered to ask if any of the charges were true. This is why my dad and I had problems. This is why I left home in the first place. My dad would not talk to me, and what I had to say never mattered. What I thought was not important. In the end the whole thing was dropped and no actual charges were ever filed against me because I was not involved.

My Dad sat there and started to dictate all the things that I would do and give up as punishment, never caring to hear what I had to say, no concern as to whether or not I had even done anything wrong or illegal. So I got up and said, "If you are not going to listen to me I will just stay here," and back to lockup I went.

Two or three hours later I was still sitting there in lockup, looking at my bunkmates for the upcoming evening, and I decided I needed to get out of there. I got the attention of a guard and asked him if he would please call my dad. I told him that I wanted to get out of here.

"Your dad is still here, he never left," the guard said. Yes, that was a big surprise to me.

As we sat down again, my dad explained to me that I was going to be grounded, that I was going to spend my days with a shovel or the jackhammer digging out the new in-ground pool in the backyard.

He also asked me to give my word that I would not just disappear like before, that I would not run away. I promised. I told myself I would stay until I'm eighteen. I would not let him run me off.

Well, I did my hard labor. I don't remember now if it was three days or three weeks, but I took his punishment and I kept my word. I did not run away. I didn't finish the pool but I gave him a really good start. But life was killing me inside. I needed to talk. I needed my dad to share thoughts and ideas with me. I was ready for more than he could allow for me.

One morning, Dad and I were in the garage and we got into an argument once again. It wasn't because I had done anything wrong, it was because I wanted to talk to him about a decision he had made. I needed to understand what he was thinking. I asked him please tell me what he was thinking. I wanted him to know that he had raised me up to be strong and independent. I wanted him to know that I had thoughts of my own. Even if he didn't agree with me I just wanted him to listen. It would make me feel like I mattered. But I got the same old, "If you live in my house you're going to live by my rules."

I explained to my father that our forefathers had left Europe to get away from tyranny. They wanted a say in their lives. That is exactly what I want… what I need. To be able to talk and discuss things that affect my life. I have never seen any person turn that red in my life and his hands were shaking. Discretion is the better part of valor, so I slowly backed away and left my dad in the garage. Our conversation was over. But all day long, I thought seriously about what he had said again about living by his rules, I realized that was fair. But this time I had promised not to disappear in the middle of the night.

It was close to midnight that day of our argument as I walked down the darkened hall. As I entered the living room I saw my dad sitting on the fireplace hearth. All he was wearing was his dingy white underwear; the color that says no one cared enough to put bleach in the laundry.

I was just barely17 years old but I felt sorry for my dad that night. I knew he was not living the life he dreamed of. I also knew he was doing his best, and he knew his best just wasn't getting it done. His marriage was over. His wife, my stepmother, had run away just like my three older sisters had. God, I never wanted to be that man.

So that night as I made my way down that dark hall, I knew what I needed to do. I asked my dad if I could talk with him, would he please just listen to me, not as his son but as a person, a man. To my surprise, he did. I explained as best I could that I could no longer live this way. I told him that I had kept my word. I did not run away, but I needed him to give me permission to go.

I tried to explain that it was because of his blood in me and how well he had raised me that I was ready to go, to be on my own, to be responsible for myself. He asked where I would go and what I would do (oh my god, he was listening to me, he was actually talking with me!). I am not sure if he was listening or if he had just given up. It doesn't matter which it was - he gave me permission to go. The next morning, when he woke up, I was gone for the last time.

I am guessing now as I look back at it, that this final gesture from him that meant so much to me was just surrender on his part. I don't really know. It was years before we spoke again.

About three years after I left home for the last time, I went back to Fresno. I visited friends including a sailing buddy and contemporary of my dad's who was also a friend of mine. After lunch with Lou and his wife Marilyn, I headed out to my truck to leave. Lou walked out with me and asked if I had been by to see my dad. I told him no. I had no reason to stop by because he didn't give a hoot about me.

Lou said you're wrong, "He carries a binder around in his truck with pictures and articles of your accomplishments in it. It's like a press book on you that he shows off to everyone he meets." I said, "Well he has never said anything to me." Then Lou said something I have never forgotten, "He will always be your dad. If you want to have a relationship, one of you is going to have to step up and be a man."

I did go by and see my dad and we did talk. It wasn't the father son talk that I had hoped for, just idle banter that he might as well have been having with someone in line at McDonalds; but we did talk.

More important is what I learned from Lou, what I want you to think about it in your life. It does not matter who is right or wrong, it does not matter who should make the move. He is my dad, I believed it was his responsibility to create and maintain a relationship with me his son!

I am an eternal optimist and on a very special day, my dad fueled my optimism. It was in the early 1990's and I had just purchased Flock-o-Matic, a light manufacturing company based in Santa Clara, California. I was living in Oregon at the time, but I was flying down every Monday morning and running the shop and crew for four, ten hour days and then flying home to Oregon every Thursday evening.

One day, just about lunch time, a car pulled up to the front door of our office/warehouse space. As the people got out of the car I was surprised to see that it was my dad and his wife, Della. After giving them the nickel tour of the facilities, my dad asked if I had time to go to lunch. I said sure, since they'd driven all the way from Fresno.

While we were at lunch, the normal limited banter about nothing in particular went on for awhile until Della kicked my dad under the table. When she kicked him, she said, "Well, aren't you going to ask him?"

My dad looked at me and asked, "Do you need help?"

WOW! I was shocked. My dad had never offered to help me with anything. He'd been doing this kind of work his whole life. I on the other hand, had no experience what so ever. A lack of experience has never stopped me from jumping into project with both feet, but to have my dad take over was terrific!

Dad's timing was perfect. My hands were tied up with other business interests and their busy seasons were fast approaching. After some discussion, Dad moved his motor home to Santa Clara and took over running the shop for me. He not only managed the crew, but he also developed a step-by-step procedure manual for the production of each item in our product line, including pictures of each step. It was an invaluable tool for future operations. My dad also used his knowledge to modify and streamline the production processes to improve the products we made and to increase our profits.

Having my dad's help lifted a large weight off my shoulders and I know that he did not do it for the money; he did it for me, his son. I had hoped that working together would be that crack in the ice of our relationship. I'm sorry to say that it wasn't. We were never able to have any discussion of a personal or emotional nature. When the job was done after a few months, my dad drove his motor home back to Fresno and that was that. What I wanted for our relationship just wasn't something my dad could give. But, he did reach out to me in the only way he could and that means the world to me. Thanks Dad!

If it is important to you… then you need to do something about it. Take the first step; take the second, heck take them all if that is what you need in your life.

Fathers and sons are known for having trouble getting along. I guess my dad and I are no different. I try to tell myself that my dad is not a bad father--that he did then and is doing now the best that he can. He raised me the best way he knew how, the way he was raised. It was near the end of an era, the principal at my grade school still had a paddle in his office and the sisters at the catholic school loved to use those rulers on my hand, corporal punishment. My dad was a product of his time. I love him and it pains my heart so that we do not have a relationship. Even more so I can't believe that he is missing out on Christopher. The couple of times that they have been together I could see how much my dad enjoyed Christopher's intelligence and interest in the things my dad was doing. They are both missing out on one of the best parts of life and it makes me so sad.

Chapter 3

Twenty years from now you will be more disappointed by the things that you didn't do than by the ones you did do. So throw off the bowlines. Sail away from the safe harbor. Catch the trade winds in your sails. Explore. Dream. Discover.

~ Mark Twain

Sometimes You Really Do
Get What You Wish For

My dad and I never really spent a lot of time together. He worked long hard hours. At the end of the day he came home completely tired, smelling like a man who'd labored all day in the hot sun. His work as a mechanical engineer had him out in the sun in California's central valley, working to repair the large equipment that the crews needed to build the dams, pave the roads and construct all sorts of buildings. During the summer months the temperature got well over 100 degrees many days. One time he showed me how the heat of the sun and the paver he was working on had burned his hands right through his thick leather gloves.

When I was about 10 years old my father said, "Come on let's go for a ride," and headed out to his truck, an old blue Chevy step side pickup. Off we went, sitting mostly in silence, with me having no idea where we were going. We went down one street turning off to another, finally turning off the main drag into a residential neighborhood.

We turned right, and then we turned left and then we headed down a street with a row of houses on each side. About halfway down the street on the left I could see a small boat upside down in somebody's yard, and as we got closer and I could see better, I realized it was a small sailboat, an El Toro. I thought to myself, "Man, wouldn't it be cool if we were here to get that boat?"

As we neared the house, my dad slowed the pickup, and to my surprise he turned into the driveway. We got out of the truck together and went over to look at the boat. I stood there inspecting it from stern to bow while my dad went to the front door and rang the doorbell.

The owner came out and we talked for a bit and then he helped us load the boat into the back of my dad's pick up. It could have been a million dollar yacht as far as I felt. I had never been so excited or as happy in my young life as I was the day my dad got me that boat.

The next day, we went to work on it. The rudder and the centerboard had not been taken care of and were in bad repair, so my dad taught me how to sand them down along with some of the woodwork inside the boat. Then he taught me how to put the marine varnish on and let me do these jobs. I have to tell you that it looked really, really nice when it was finished and it felt good to have done that work with my own two hands. That boat looked brand new.

The first weekend after the repairs were done, we loaded the boat up into the truck and we took it to the lake. My dad helped me put the mast in place, showed me how to raise the sail, rig all the rigging with the main sheet, the outhaul and the boomerang. He explained to me how it all worked, put me in the boat and shoved me off from the shore. I remember looking back my dad standing on the shore as I sailed further and further away from him and I wondered how I was going to do this. In the first few minutes I felt a mixture of excitement and fear. But my fear quickly gave way to the excitement, as my mind went back to those many weekends and most of our family vacations watching my dad and helping him on our family sailboat. I had nothing to fear. I was the captain of my own ship!

The excitement of sailing your own boat, the wind blowing in your face, the water slapping on the hull, is something that you don't appreciate unless you have actually experienced it. As a young boy, it meant more to me than anything else I had done.

My dad had picked out that boat, he'd taught me how to refinish it, and he'd shown his confidence in me by shoving me off the shore – sink or swim, baby – and swim I did.

The El Toro was just the first of many sailboats my dad got for me as I worked my way up to a couple of bigger boats, and I soon became involved in racing. My dad was a member of the Fresno Yacht Club where they had regattas most weekends, and some midweek evenings all through the spring, summer and fall. My sailboat-racing career began in that El Toro and then I moved up to other boats including the Laser, the Force Five, the Lido, the Day Sailor, Thistles, Catalina 22's, and others. I sailed freshwater lakes, rivers and offshore racing.

Sailboat racing was a lot of fun; meeting the new people and having a sense of freedom. Because of the lessons my dad had taught me and an awful lot of luck, I brought home trophies on a regular basis and it felt good to be recognized for winning.

Because of my success, I was invited to help other people in racing. One such opportunity was a trip to San Francisco Bay to race the 470, a lightweight boat, and extremely fast. The boat was mostly open – the design was such that you spent almost no time on the hull. Most of the time my feet were on the edge of the boat and I wore a harness and was attached to the top of the mast by a cable called a trapeze. I spent the vast majority of my time out on this trapeze screaming across the water as fast as a sailboat could go.

As luck would have it, while racing the 470 in the San Francisco Bay area, one of the shrouds broke and we lost the mast. The boat capsized and my racing partner Michael and I were in the water. Michael was trapped underneath the mainsail. I got him out from underneath and we held on to that hull. We quickly learned the meaning of the word hypothermia. By the time the rescue boat got to us, we had already seen the fin of a shark, and apparently we were turning blue. I also learned that the best remedy for hypothermia is for someone who is nice and warm to strip off all his or her clothes and cuddle up next to you to share body heat. That was a strange experience for a young boy of just 14. I did not know the woman on the boat who rescued my fellow sailor Michael and me out of the water. I did learn that she wore a bra and panties with very strange patterns that did not match as she snuggled up to me as we were wrapped in a blanket.

Another time we were racing in the Catalina 22 Nationals off of Southern California. I had a very strange and eerie feeling. I looked over my left shoulder and all I could see was a wall of green water. It was what is referred to as a "rogue wave." As I hugged myself close to the bulkhead at the entryway to the cabin, the wave crashed down on the boat. The wave knocked the boat down, tore the mast off, and knocked some of the crew overboard. This was a very, very scary event and it taught me my first lesson about the strength and the danger of the ocean. Everyone was rescued and was in good health but that fear is forever etched in my mind.

As I think about all of the places sailing has taken me, and all the fun I have had as a youngster and as I have grown older sailing around the world, I think back fondly to that evening my dad said, "Come on, let's go for a ride," and the excitement that welled up inside of me as I dreamed about getting that boat I saw down the street – knowing full well that there was no way that boat was for me. My dad surprised me that evening, and it changed by life in a big way, in a very positive way.

As I look back at my life, there are not a lot of positive things that come to mind about my childhood. But my dad teaching me to sail, teaching me to race sailboats and giving me the opportunity to travel, are some of my fondest and most exciting memories.

Speaking of excitement reminds me of a time in Colorado in the early 1980's. I had a Laser, a 14' one-man boat, and I took it to Dillon Reservoir way up in the Rocky Mountains by the Keystone Ski Resort. By the time I got there a storm was starting to blow in over the mountains, and I could see the skies darkening and the whitecaps picking up all across the lake. As far as you could see, boats were heading in.

But I am a heavy weather sailor – the stronger the wind the better. I can't stand calm seas. So I rigged up the Laser, pushed off from shore, and off I went. The wind was blowing so hard, the whitecaps were breaking, half the time I couldn't tell if I was above the water or below it as the waves broke across my face.

About halfway across the lake, I came across a large keelboat, a Catalina 25 coming in from the far side. They had their jib down and their main sail furled for the heavy weather. I heard the Captain exclaim, as he saw me hooting and hollering, having the time of my life, "God, I wish I could be doing that."

The one thing that stuck in my mind, other than what a great time I was having, was that I never, ever in my life wanted to be that guy. The guy who says, "Gee, I wish I could be doing that. Gosh, I wish I were having the fun they are having." I never wanted to be that guy, and I've worked hard my entire life to make sure I never was.

Chapter 4

One-half of life is luck; the other half is discipline - and that's the important half, for without discipline you wouldn't know what to do with luck.

~ Carl Zuckmeyer

Winning the Lottery!

It was about 11 PM on a Friday night and they were prepared to do the drawing for the Colorado lottery, $12,500,000 was the prize that night. I was lying in bed watching the drawing on TV. They called the first number, and lo and behold I had it. Then they called the second number, I had that one too. Not much to get excited about though, I'm not yet in the money. Then they called the third number and I had it. Three bucks - not bad for a one-dollar investment.

But I was looking for more, much more …$12,500,000 to be exact. I am sitting up in bed when they call the fourth number. I had it. Now I'm a little bit more excited, and I'm standing on the bed. They call the fifth number and I've got it too. So now not only am I standing on the bed; I am jumping up-and-down a little bit because I'm only one number away from the grand prize. And then as I stare at the screen I see them select number 41 and am jumping up and down on the bed… I am so excited, $12,500,000! I am hooting and hollering and jumping up and down, I just can't believe it… I am the winner.

They called number 41 and I HAVE IT . . . Yaa Hooo! As I had a chance to relax and calm down I looked at the ticket again, they had called number 41… I had number 14.

I called a friend in California to commiserate that I had just won, and then lost, the Colorado lottery for $12,500,000. But he told me that 5 out of 6 was a guaranteed $100,000. Furthermore, he said, it's $100,000 when the prize is only $1,000,000 and yours was $12,500,000, which means you probably are going to get $1,250,000.

So I thought okay I did not win $12,500,000 but $1,250,000 is nothing to sneeze at. The next morning I went down to the local King Soopers store where I bought the ticket and had them scan it. Sure enough the lady said "Your ticket is a winner, so much money that we can't pay you here, you're going to have to go to the lottery office." I'm starting to feel pretty good again. No jumping up and down but I'm feeling pretty good. All Saturday night and all day Sunday I waited.

Monday morning I jumped into my car and headed to the lottery office. When I got there I presented my lottery ticket and the nice lady at the counter scanned it. She said, "Sure enough it's a winner; I need to see a photo ID and a social security card." I provided her with both. Then she went away to print the check. When she got back she slid the check under the glass to me, I took a quick look at it and I said, "Nope" and slid it right back to her under the glass. She opened it up, took a look at it and slid it right back to me. I picked it up and looked at it again and I said. "No . . . 5 out of 6 that's a guaranteed $100,000." She shook her head.

The lady was kind enough to explain that in *California,* 5 out of 6 is a guaranteed $100,000 minimum payment. But this is Colorado she reminded me, here we do things a little bit different. I opened up the check, looked at it again. And I will tell you that it was the first time in my life that I've ever been angry, truly angry that someone had given me $631!

From Drop Out to Guru

Chapter 5

I do those things which seem correct to me today. I trust myself. And if security concerns me, I do that which today I think will make me secure. And every day I do that, and when that day arrives that I need a reserve,(a)odds are that I have it, and (b) the true reserve that I have is the strength that I have of acting each day without fear.

~ Anonymous

My Life in Work – A Summary

Some people spend their whole life in one job or on a single career path. That did not really work for me. I wanted to learn new skills; to develop new talents that I could bring to whatever project came next in my life.

One of the businesses that I worked in was the Reforestation Industry. It mainly involves replanting where areas have been logged and after natural disasters like a forest fire and even after volcanoes, like the work that was done on Mount Saint Helens after she blew her top. It also includes pre-commercial thinning and trail maintenance. External factors such as frozen ground and snowed over roads caused the reforestation business to be seasonal. The seedlings would freeze and die before you could get them in the ground in the winter months.

In the summer months the heat and lack of moisture would bring on an unacceptably high level of mortality for the seedlings planted. There was also an extreme fire danger in the forests at that time of year, dramatically restricting the ability to work. That meant two or three months in the spring and then another two to three months in the fall and our work was done for the year.

At first this seemed like the perfect schedule, make a boat load of money and then get three months off to spend it. I admit it was fun for a while, but it did not take long for me to get bored. Only so much skiing, fishing, camping, and hiking I could do and then my brain started begging for stimulation. Give me a challenge, something new to learn.

That is where a lot of these professions listed below came from, during the summer doing this and during the winter doing that. A handful of these demand more than just a spot on some list so I have written more in later chapters for a few. But to go into complete detail on each and everyone would take a whole different book all to itself.

Job's I've held:

Paper Boy * Hamburger Stand Employee * Sailing Instructor *
Potato Harvester * Thinning Crew * Tree Planter (Reforestation) *
Standup Comedian * Framer * Roofer * Electrical System Installer
* Real Estate Investor * Trainer for Rent-a-Center * Promoter -
50's Rock 'n' Roll and Vaudeville shows * Consultant for Weapons
Corporation of America * Sales Trainer/Motivational Speaker *
Corporate Consultant for We Care America * Adjunct Professor of
Law * Speech Coach and Inspirational/Motivational Speaker *

Businesses I've owned:

* National Legal Shield (Prepaid legal) * Diversified
Administrators, Inc. * National Marketing Consultants * Christmas
Tree Lots * Lock Protector * Christmas Tree Farm * Churchill
Enterprises, Inc. * oregonsbestwine.com * Vineyard Supply busi-
ness * Creative Real Estate Development * Someday Group *

Chapter 6

Expecting life to treat you well because you are a good person is like expecting an angry bull not to charge because you are a vegetarian.

~ Shari R. Barr

The Trust of a Stranger

I was working on a tree planting crew out of Brookings, Oregon. The foreman was a rather cagey fellow by the name of Jako Jako. (Yes, that really was his name!) It was hard physical work. The units (areas mapped out by the forest service where the work was to be done) were very steep, covered with slash, and most of the time it was raining and cold. There were 11 Mexicans and one seventeen year old white boy, me, working on the crew with Jako as foreman.

Most evenings after work, our crew and other crews in the area would wind up in the Chetco Inn, the main drinking establishment in the area. Because of his rather unique and somewhat undesirable physical features, Jako had a little more trouble with the women than he wished. So one evening he struck upon a great idea, and after finding himself what they call being "three sheets to the wind" he headed to a local jewelry store. It did not seem to bother him that it was closed and after-hours. He broke in, gathered up as much jewelry as he could hold in his pockets and in his hands and came back to the Chetco Inn. He explained to the attractive young cocktail waitress that she could have her pick of any of his fine treasures if she would spend time with him.

Sober Jako wasn't real subtle, and drunk he was extremely loud. So most everybody in the bar knew what he was doing, and most folks could figure out how he was accomplishing this task. It didn't take long for a few uniformed police officers to show up at the Chetco Inn and take Jako Jako away, for some free room and board at the county jail.

With our foreman in jail, the crew was leaderless, so the contractor that we were all working for came down from Hood River. His name was Aaron Curtis, a bear of a man from Alaska originally. Aaron's favorite phrase was "Hurry every chance you get" and regardless of how distasteful his projects were, he would always tell you that, "It was better than a jab in the eye with a sharp stick."

Well, Mr. Curtis came to the hotel to talk with me. He said, "You're the only person on the crew with a drivers license, how would you like to be the new foreman?" I asked, "What does that entail?" He replied, "Instead of making eight dollars an hour you'll be getting 25% of the profits." This sounded like a whole lot better deal for me, so I signed up to be foreman.

Now that I was a new member of the upper class in reforestation, a newly minted foreman, the other foreman let me sit and talk with them. I quickly learned that my 25% of profits was below the industry standard. Another contractor took notice of the performance of my crew and offered me the opportunity to run a crew for him on another job after Brookings. Once my commitment on the Brookings job was done, I would start working with the other contractor and earn 40% of profits on the new job. There was one condition; the new job required that I have my own pickup truck in order to carry all the tools that were necessary to complete the job.

This was all good news except for the fact that I did not have a pickup truck. I didn't have a car at the time and was relying on the crummy (the crew rig, full of all those sweaty men and all of their trash, day after day) for transportation from the hotel to the job site and from job to job. When the Brookings job was done, I returned home to Bend, Oregon and proceeded to look for a truck.

In the local paper I found several trucks advertised. I narrowed it down to a Ford truck that had a camper shell that could be locked, thereby protecting the tools. But the problem was the owner wanted $3,500 for it. I only had about $1,000 saved up. I explained to my sister Bonnie, what I wanted to do. She agreed to drive me over to look at the truck and give me an opportunity to talk to the owner

After Bonnie and I looked over the truck and took it for a test drive, we decided that it would definitely suit my needs. And so I sat down with the owner and I explained my circumstances. I told him the work that I had been doing and what I was getting paid. I explained to him that I had become a foreman. I even told him about Jako Jako, and how I got the job. It was a funny story… and he laughed. Then I explained to him that I began work as a foreman at 25%. Now, I had an opportunity to work as a foreman for 40% on new job in the Ashland, Oregon area, but that I needed to have a truck. I explained to him that I liked his truck and it would do the job, but I just didn't have all the money. And what I would like for him to do was take my thousand dollars as a down payment and let me take his truck to the job. In a few weeks when the job was over I would come back and pay off the balance of the truck.

This man did not know me from Adam in a group of two! He had talked to me for a while. He heard my stories and met my sister. When I asked him that question, he looked me up and down sizing me up. Then he stuck out his hand and he said some words that have stuck with me to this day… **"Don't let me down."**

I don't think a young man has ever been more excited and giddy and happy and hooting and hollering than I was that day when I drove away in my new truck. I was riding high on the faith and trust of a stranger.

When the job was over, I returned to this man with the balance of the money for the truck. There was not an ounce of surprise in his expression as I showed up with the rest of his money, and I did my best to communicate to him how much it meant to me that he trusted me and gave me the opportunity to improve my life. It is decades later and I still remember that day.

Unfortunately I don't remember his name, but I hope that if he is still alive that he will read this book. If he does, he will know how much it meant to me. If he told this story to some his family and any of them read this book, please get in touch with me. I'd like to tell them face-to-face. And if not, I want them to know that funny story he told them about that boy and his truck, meant a whole lot more to me than they could ever imagine.

Chapter 7

Laugh when you can, apologize when you should, and let go of what you can't change. Kiss slowly, play hard, forgive quickly, take chances, give everything and have no regrets. Life's too short to be anything...but happy.

~ Author Unknown

Silver Dollar Bar at the Wort Hotel

It was very late on a Saturday night in Jackson Hole, Wyoming. We had all been working long days on the other side of the Tetons near the town of Driggs, Idaho. We were working to complete a thinning job for the forest service. Thinning is where you work your way through a marked area of the forest and remove specified trees to allow the remaining trees to grow to their best potential.

This job was complicated by a lack of sleep brought on by two things. First, because we were behind on the schedule, we were working long days. We would start just after sunrise early in the morning and work up to about ten hours each day, depending on where each unit would end. Ten hours of hard and dangerous work and then we headed back to camp for a dinner break. Once dinner was done we would head back to the unit, and you guessed it, another four or five hours of manhandling our chain saws. Then back to camp where we would fall into our sleeping bags totally exhausted.

Fourteen to fifteen hours a day fighting the slash, the mountain and that dammed man-eating saw. Under any circumstances this schedule would have been tough, but we were working on a thinning job. That means each and every member of the crew was climbing up and down the mountainsides, over slash piles, the whole while dealing with a chainsaw that could eat you alive. It is scary how fast a chain saw can go through human flesh and bone. I witnessed way too many accidents but the one that stands out in my mind was crazy Dave. I never knew his real name as everybody on the crew just called him crazy Dave.

One day late in the afternoon while we were working, I heard a blood-curdling scream. It was so loud I heard it over the sound of my own chain saw. I let go of the throttle and looked back over my shoulder. There was crazy Dave with his chainsaw running full throttle, whipping around over his head. That scream was coming from him. As I looked down I saw blood pouring out from where his kneecap used to be. He had walked into his saw while it was running. We wanted to help him but that saw was whipping about his head. We were afraid that he would cut himself again and us as well if we approached him. So everybody was hollering at Dave to drop the saw… "Dave just drop the saw!!!" Finally he did and we were able to get pressure on his wound and transport him down the mountain to the hospital. The hair on my arms stands up as I write about this with the memory of that blood-curdling scream still ringing in my ears.

The second reason was far more stressful. Several nights during this job we were visited by grizzly bears, eight feet tall and 750 pounds. We were all in tents which provided no protection, when they wanted in they got in. Ice chests were destroyed and a dog was killed. Going with the safety in numbers idea some of us bunked together. My sister and brother-in-law along with their two young boys agreed to let me move me into their large, family style tent.

One evening my brother-in-law Dan, and I awoke to the sound of a bear moving ever closer to our tent. Both of us were armed, my rifle was a lever action 30/30 and Dan had a 30.06 bolt action hunting rifle. After listening carefully, Dan and I decided that the bear was about 200 feet away near the road. I handed my 30/30 to Dan so I could unzip the tent, all of the sudden I heard BLAM, BLAM, BLAM!!! I think my ears are still ringing . . . The bear was not at the road as we had thought. He was just outside the tent about 30 feet away. As the tent flap opened and the light of the Coleman lantern reached outside, Dan saw the bear and from a kneeling position ripped off several rounds from my 30/30 about two feet from my ears.

The grizzly bear rose up, made a furious noise then spun and ran up the slope to the road and into the night. There was no sleep to be had for the rest of the night. We just knew in our hearts that the bear was coming back to get us. At first light we found a blood trail and tracked him for over an hour, but we lost the trail and never found that bear. For the next few days everyone on the job was watching over their shoulders a little more than normal.

Sleep never came easy on that job, and we looked forward to our breaks in the big city, Jackson Hole. As for the bear problem we found out that it was a classic example of the left hand not knowing what the right hand was doing . . . The problem bears from Yellowstone were being relocated to a drop site about 5 miles from our camp!

As for our weekend in the big city we were going to blow off some steam and take in a show and see a country music non-super-star, Rusty Draper.

Saturday night found us taking in a comedy show at the Silver Dollar Bar at the Wort Hotel. The crowd was well lubed up with alcohol by the time the comedian took the stage. It did not take long for the crowd to decide that this guy was nowhere near funny, not even sure he had ever been close to funny. About fifteen minutes into his act the crowd started to voice their displeasure. It was starting to get ugly and then all of the sudden I heard a voice coming out of me, "Hey buddy, do you know what a microphone is?" He looked at the one in his hand and said yea. I said, "Why don't you do us all a favor and . . ." OK, I was younger and did not have the filter that I do now!

The crowd went crazy with laughter, and he said, "Well if you think you can do better, why don't you come up here and give it a try?" Remember when I said the crowd was well lubed up for the show . . . I guess I had consumed just enough to make me think that his invitation was a good idea. So to the thunderous applause of the crowd, up to the stage I went. This was despite the wishes of my date and several of my family members.

The crowd was going wild as I made my way to the stage, I turned around to face my audience and all I saw was a row of cowboy boots poking out of the darkness. Having never been on a stage before, I was surprised to find that I could not see that loving audience I was hoping to connect with. The very bright spotlights shining on me prevented me from seeing the audience. For a split second I was not sure what was going to happen, was I going to freeze, could I remember any jokes?

Hey, my job was to help get him off the stage, not to get me on it. So I gave the audience a couple of simple jokes that I could re-member, the audience went crazy again. Lucky for me the guy was sooo bad and the audience was drunk enough to laugh at anything and everything I said. I relaxed when I realized I could have said, "blue bucket" and they would have laughed at it. I ripped off three or four more jokes and left the stage to thunderous applause. People were slapping me high fives all the way back to my table.

Once there, several people came up to me, some said how good I was; some said it was a set up, that I had sent the first guy up to make my act look good. A few very nice ladies came over and asked me to dance; that did not make my date happy, even though I turned them all down.

So one crazy night during 1977 in the Silver Dollar Bar at The Wort Hotel in Jackson Hole WY I got to add yet another job to my resume . . . Standup Comedian.

Chapter 8

Life is a succession of lessons which must be lived to be understood.

~ Helen Keller

Who is Everett?

The simplest answer is Everett is my brother-in-law. He is married to my middle sister Bonnie. They have been married since I was in grade school, a long-term relationship by any measurement.

But Everett is more to me than just a brother-in-law. Everett taught me a lot about business, but more importantly, he taught me about life. As a young teenager who struck out on his own, there was so much I didn't know. It was Everett who filled in many of the gaps.

I remember one day in Bend, Oregon, hanging out with some friends sitting on their couch. I was reading a magazine and enjoying some good music. It was a nice enough day, but emotionally I wasn't feeling that well. And then there came a knock at the door. Jean, the lady of the house answered the door and then she came into the living room and said, "David, it is for you." I was surprised because I wasn't expecting company, and I wasn't sure that anybody actually knew I was there. I went to the door, it was Everett. He wasn't mad, he wasn't happy; he was just there to talk to me.

You see, I was running a crew on a job that Everett's company had contracted with the forest service to complete. Because of some personal problems that I was having, I had decided not to go to work that day. Everett asked me what I was doing. He asked me if I was okay, if I was sick. I explained to Everett, that I was not sick. I was just dealing with these personal problems and didn't feel like going to work that day.

Everett explained that it wasn't just about me. He explained to me that there was an entire crew of men who were unable to earn their wages that day, simply because I decided not to go to work. An entire crew of men who were paying hotel bills that day, but not earning any money. He reminded me that there was a contractual time limit to complete the job, and that by taking unplanned days off I had put the entire job in jeopardy. Everett's company was at risk of being defaulted for failing to complete the job in a timely fashion.

He said he understood problems in general and that he understood emotional problems specifically. He said he understood a lot of things, but he didn't understand how one person could make a decision that would negatively impact so many others without giving it more consideration.

Hey, I was at the end of my teenage years and he was right, thoughts about those other people never crossed my mind. He said, "David, you're a man now, and you can make whatever choice you want to make. But you need to understand that every choice you make from this point forward in your life has consequences. Not just consequences for you, but consequences for other people as well. So I hope that tomorrow, you and your crew are back on the job doing the top-notch job that I have come to expect and rely on. But the choice is truly yours."

Yes, we were on the job the next day. Were my personal problems resolved, no. But I found the distraction of work actually helped.

Everett gave me a new way of looking at things, a lesson that has stuck with me all these years: We are intertwined, what we do has consequences . . . beyond just ourselves.

There was a time, early in my career, that I went to Everett to explain that I needed capital to take advantage of a business opportunity. Not just any business opportunity but a great business opportunity, one that would have huge returns, and all I needed was $10,000 and I could make millions!

Everett made me a very simple offer; he said he would give me the $10,000 that I needed. If I was sure that this deal would guarantee millions of dollars of income in the long run he would give me that money. All I had to do to get the seed money was to sign over 50% of my future earnings to him. Well to those of us who are adults now that seems kind of onerous. And to those who are familiar with The Colonel will remember that he got 50% of everything Elvis earned. Elvis and his family have lived quite well on that 50%. I guess that was the point Everett was trying to make, or was it?

I took my time to think about this offer and to think about things

I had learned from Everett. I believe the lesson he was trying to teach me was that we have to think about the long-term value of what we're doing today. Today, it's we have to have this or we have to do that. It seems that way, but that's not always the case. When you take the time to think about what the long-term effects really will be of the decisions we make today, we make better decisions.

Nope, I did not take Everett up on his offer of $10,000 for half of my future income. Man what a good deal that would've been for Everett. And even though I knew at that time that I **needed** that money, I **had** to do that deal. It wasn't true, and for the rest of my life, I was very happy that I did not take the money and took the time to think it through.

I've tried to think of a story that would best sum up this next lesson. There are just too many of them. Not one stands above the others so great that it should be included and the others not, so let me just tell you what I learned. It's a real simple truth.

"A man is only as good as his word."

Generations ago, everybody believed this, but it's gotten lost. And I think it's a shame, a shame for our society as a whole and for individuals as well. There are other ways to say it. "Say what you mean, mean what you say." "Do what you say." But it all boils down to the fact that it's true. A man is only as good as his word. It's important to me that my friends, my family, and people that I do business with can trust that what I tell them is true. If I make a promise or commitment, I'm going to stick with it. They can count on me.

One day back in the early eighties my nephew Roger made a comment to Everett, that I was so lucky. Everett replied to him that I was lucky because I made my own luck. That comment has stayed with me over the years. It is something that I would like you to do to… make your own luck. Look for the positive in each situation; be prepared to cash in on every opportunity that comes your way. Be open to new roads and new ideas. Make your own luck!

Thank you… Everett… I owe you a debt I can never repay.

Chapter 9

Above all, challenge yourself. You may well surprise yourself at what strengths you have, what you can accomplish.

~ Cecile M. Springer

Where Did You Get Your J.D.?

Having left home at such an early age, I had failed to complete high school. Not graduating from high school didn't leave room for attending college. But life's strange turns and circumstances, which so often for me become opportunities, allowed me to teach college. Here is a story about one of those turns in life.

I was introduced to the concept of prepaid legal plans in Bend, Oregon in the late seventies. A man named Don Caldwell from Sacramento, California invented the concept. He had a great idea, but lacked the ability to successfully market it. A lesson learned over and over again in my life, good ideas are a dime a dozen. The value is in that someone who can get it done.

Upon reviewing the concept and seeing a great opportunity, I decided that someone to get it done would be me. So I created a plan and successfully built the business across the country.

With National Legal Shield, the main company I built in this industry, people could get a plan for themselves as an individual or family, or a business plan for commercial needs and we offered employee benefit plans to be provided to employees by their employer. All of National Legal Shield's plans allowed people to get quality legal services at a cost that they could afford.

My work and success in developing the new industry of prepaid legal plans got me noticed locally and then nationally by a lot of different associations and media outlets.

National TV shows, radio shows and different publications were listing me as an expert in the field of prepaid legal plans. The media christened me "The Guru of Prepaid Legal." My leadership position in the field gave me an opportunity to speak to many different associations and groups, including the American Bar Association.

In order to maintain their law licenses, attorneys are required to have a certain number of continuing legal education (CLE) hours annually. So when Denver University decided that it wanted to offer a course on prepaid legal plans as part of its CLE program, who better to call on than The Guru of Prepaid Legal? That is how I got to work as an Adjunct Professor at Denver University College of Law, or DU.

DU had contacted the American Bar Association to get a teaching reference for their CLE program on Prepaid Legal. After receiving the referral, a representative of DU called me in order to put the course syllabus together. The nice lady on the phone confirmed my name and address and then she asked, "Where did you get your J.D.?"

I said I didn't have a J.D., and there was a long pause. Truth be told, when she asked that question I had no idea what a J.D. was, I just knew I didn't have one.

She then asked, "Well, where did you graduate college?"

I replied that I had never graduated from college. There was a much longer pause. Guess it's a good thing I didn't tell her that I had never even attended any college.

Then just as I began to think her pause would never end, she asked, "Do I have the right David A. Koop?"

After my long explanation and I am sure a few behind the scenes phone calls on her part, the syllabus was completed. The courses were well attended and well received.

That's right, I have never attended college but I have taught college as an Adjunct Professor of Law at Denver University College of Law. Don't let the lack of formal training hold you back, do what you want to do.

Yes, I found out what a J.D. was - a Juris Doctorate, fancy name for a law degree.

Chapter 10

Whatever you want in life, start today.
Not tomorrow - today.
Let it be a small beginning - a tiny beginning.
Your happiness depends on starting today - every day.

~ Jonathan Lockwood Huie

Churchill Enterprises, Inc.

Most people, after hearing my explanation of my business life respond with one of two thoughts… "Oh, like Monopoly, just with real money" or "You're like Richard Gere in Pretty Woman."

What I did for most of my adult life was buy and sell companies. I would find the right small and medium sized company and buy it. Companies whose operations had stayed in the stone age, companies whose owners were ready to retire or whose owners were good idea people but did not like or were no good at building the company. Normally these owners had not modernized their business, and had not taken advantage of technology or leveraging their own brand or customer relationships.

I would work hard to maximize profits through the use of new technologies and brand leveraging. These improvements in the business would normally allow the acquisition to pay for itself. I also looked for competitors and prime vendors that we could acquire and roll up to take advantage of the economies of scale.

The best example of this strategy was a small company based in South San Francisco, by the San Francisco International Airport and the massive Bay Area UPS hub (a fact that we would capitalize on to raise our competitive advantage).

The company, Churchill Enterprises, was started in 1947 by Howard and Betty Churchill. It started out as a hardware store. I know this not only from them telling me but because I became the lucky owner of some of their carryover stock from the long closed hardware store.

Around the time of World War II, they started selling Christmas trees. Over the years as more and more profits were derived from the short Christmas season, the hardware store went by the wayside and selling Christmas trees and the supplies needed for running a Christmas tree lot became the focus of Churchill.

They were no longer just retailing trees, but also developing a tree wholesaling business. The hard goods for retailers were growing right along with it. Eventually retail supplies came to outpace the retail and wholesale tree side. Everything that a lot owner would need to sell Christmas trees: stands, flock, flocking machines, tags, banners, flame retardant, tree preservative and much more. Churchill's business grew to generate a low six-figure income with the benefit of only a few weeks of work for the season.

At the time I started my due diligence (investigating all facets of the business as presented to me) the supply side was operating out of a warehouse shared with a small sheet metal business and the wholesale yard for trees was about five blocks away. The business had no computers, everything was done by hand. Customer lists, customer records, inventory, invoicing and billing all done by hand. On each desk, buried under stacks of 3 x 5 cards and papers, were two separate rotary phones. No multiline phone systems with hold, or paging and intercom features, no extensions anywhere out in the warehouse.

When we finally did close the sale and all of the 3 x 5 customer cards were turned over, more than 20% were so badly written that none of the sellers or anyone on my team could decipher the important customer details. Opportunities lost to the old ways.

My next purchase was Flock-O-Matic, the patent holder for the best flocking machines in the industry. One of Churchill's prime vendors was now integrated into our company. The end of Churchill's second season saw the closure of the wholesale yard. The separate expenses for rent, phones, payroll, and the cost of rental trucks and the lack of reliable drivers for delivery all around the Bay Area did not pencil out. Not as compared to our new alternative delivery system that our increased volume allowed us to command. Because of our large volume we could deliver fresher trees, direct from the farms in Oregon with customer orders as small as 150 trees.

Orders with the original delivery trucks as set up by Churchill were either 150 or 300 trees (half a load or a full load). So the only business we lost was the very small handful of retail storeowners who came in for 15 to 25 trees at a time from the wholesale yard. The cost savings and the reduced liability were massive.

Next came the acquisition of GreenerN'ever, a competitor of Churchill's based in the Monterey Bay area. A year later, I acquired Bing Enterprises, another wholesale supply company based in Chicago Illinois, serving customers nationwide, but mainly in the Midwest. The last major acquisition involving Churchill was The Christmas Company. Based in Oxnard, California, this was yet another competitor of Churchill's with customers nationwide, but mainly serving the Southern California area.

During the years of acquisitions, we started our private label products to brand our place in the market. Some of the main products included Flock-O-Matic the Christmas tree flock, since we owned the Flock-O-Matic line of machines. The GreenerN'ever name was used to brand many products including our tree preservative and flame retardant products. Rolling all of these competitors and vendors into Churchill benefited us in several ways. We got dramatic economies of scale; reduction of overlapping cost on staff, facilities, advertising, travel and booth cost for a series of national and local trade shows.

Also the increased volume allowed us to lower our product cost across the line with our vendors and the removal of competitors in the marketplace helped to achieve optimal pricing. Lots of years having fun acquiring and building the business traveling the country as it threw off profits to allow me to enjoy life.

Churchill was included in that "Get your affairs in order" directive that I got. I was able to sell the company just prior to the 2006 season and focus on my fight with cancer as well as building memories with Christopher.

Chapter 11

When you were born, you cried and the world rejoiced. Live your life so that when you die, the world cries and you rejoice.

~ Cherokee Expression

Christopher

"Look at those hands, they're huge!"

As I heard those words I stood up from the head of the operating table where my wife, Elaine, was having an emergency C-section. That is when I saw my son for the first time. He was wailing away creating quite a racket. Because of the concern at the end of the pregnancy, our pediatrician was there. He and two of the nurses in the operating room quickly took our new son over to a separate table to do the APGAR score and to ensure that he was okay.

This was not supposed to be happening on this day. You see Christopher's mom was an attorney who practiced family law. During the late term of her pregnancy, I would put on my three-piece suit and tie and carried her trial case for her as she continued to practice law. We had a regularly scheduled appointment with Dr. Case, our OB/GYN. So we stopped there on our way to a court appearance that day. It was supposed to be a regular checkup. But when they placed the fetal heart monitor on Elaine's ever-growing tummy, it was apparent even to a layperson that something was not quite right. Regular beat, regular beat and then it dropped off. Not a good feeling.

I could actually see our son's heart distress on the monitor and closing my eyes did not help as I could hear the beep, beep, beep . . . pause then beep again, over and over. I held Elaine's hand and told her everything would be OK.

The nurse came in and read the tape printout from the monitor and said she'd be right back, as she quickly left the room. Moments later, Dr. Case came in and read the tape from the fetal heart monitor. Dr. Case explained to us that our baby's heart was in distress, and that they were going to induce labor, right then.

Pitocin was injected, and we began the process of induced labor. Dr. Case's office was in the hospital, so all of this transpired very fast. Attempts were made for a normal delivery, but Christopher just did not want to come out. Finally, between Christopher refusing to come out and his distress on the monitor increasing, the doctors decided that Elaine should undergo an emergency C-section. This brings me back to that racket in the room…

Christopher was wailing away the whole time they were checking him out. Finally, the pediatrician asked if I wanted to come and see our son. As I walked over, he continued wailing to the best of his ability. Who knew a newborn child could make such a racket?

As I got to the table I moved in between the two nurses, leaned slightly forward and said, "Hello Christopher." He immediately stopped crying and rolled his head in my direction and locked his gaze onto me, silent as he could be.

Our pediatrician said, "Man, does he track on your voice." During the pregnancy I regularly talked to our son, told him stories and sang songs to him. I think what the experts say is true, kids can hear you in the womb. Christopher could pick my voice out from all others in the room.

After they swaddled him in his blanket they asked if I would like to hold him. I melted in his gaze as I held him close. I moved over to the head of the operating table and introduced Christopher to his mom.

While surgeons finished with Elaine, Christopher and I moved to our birthing room, and I got to give him his first bath. I was so happy, so proud, and so scared. I was scared that I might break him, all the while being dazed by the wonderment of it all.

To this day I still carry the photo of his first bath in my wallet. I have had many great days in my life doing a lot of different and wonderful things. But this was and still is, the most amazing day of my life, and yet, it was also the beginning of a dark time in my life.

I wish I could tell you that Christopher's birth was a miracle – an immaculate conception! But we all know, that wouldn't be true. I had waited my entire life for a family, for a true partner and great woman by my side and for children. I thought I'd found her in Christopher's mom.

We were actually introduced by our dentist. I was a new patient and it was my first visit to the dental office. So of course the dental assistants were chattier than usual because they were trying to find out about the new patient.

When they asked what I had been doing I explained that I had been unloading boxes for the last few days, because I had just moved into a big new house up on the hill. The hygienist replied, "Your wife must be very excited." I said, "No, because I don't have a wife, but I am taking applications." The two female dental assistants both laughed.

The rest of the appointment went on without a hitch. I got a full exam and got my teeth cleaned. With the appointment completed, I was out the door with my bag of samples and a new toothbrush.

I headed back to my new house on the hill, changed back into grungys and proceeded to empty yet another box. About an hour to an hour and a half later my phone rang. I answered the phone and was surprised to find the receptionist from the dentist office on the line. She said, "Hi David, I hope this isn't inappropriate but I was thinking about what you said about accepting applications for a wife."

I thought for sure she was going to ask me out. I was thinking, oh man how do I get out of this one? The receptionist seemed to be nice enough the two minutes that I got to speak with her in the office, but she just was not the sort of woman I would date.

My breathing went back to normal as she let me off the hook, she said, "We have a patient that I think would be great for you. She is from Canada and is very beautiful. Would it be OK if we give her your number?" I said sure. The receptionist asked me hold on for just a minute. When she came back on the line she said that she had given my number to their patient and that their patient had asked them to share her number with me.

The receptionist asked if I would call this woman if they gave me her number, I said yes I would. She asked yet again are you sure that you will call? I repeated that yes I would, as I said, I would call her. She then told me that her name was Elaine, and she is very pretty she told me once again and then she gave me her number. With that behind me I went back to work unpacking boxes.

After giving up on the boxes in favor of dinner I noticed the note with the phone number on it. I wondered how long I should wait to give her a call, one day, three days, so many published and unpublished rules about how the game is supposed to work. I have never been one for games or rules so I decided to give her a call right then.

I dialed the number and shortly there was an answer, a female voice said hello. I introduced myself and asked if she was Elaine, sure enough I had made contact with the very pretty lady from Canada. We made small talk for a while and then I asked if she would like to get together sometime for coffee or maybe dinner and she said yes! We set a date and place for drinks.

When I got to the door I told the hostess that I was to meet a young lady there, she told me that my date was waiting for me in the bar. As she turned to lead me to where Elaine was waiting she said, "She is very pretty." There was that statement yet again and I begin to wonder if she was paying people to say that about her.

As we got to the bar I got my first look at Elaine and realized that she did not need to pay anyone to make nice comments about her. She was waiting at a booth and I joined her for what was to be a drink before she headed out of town. We talked with ease for quite awhile and the plan for just a drink turned into dinner. Both of us left the restaurant that night with smiles on our faces.

Frequent and serious dating commenced right away and our relationship flourished. Elaine was all I was looking for in a partner, or so I thought: smart, funny, playful and flirtatious. The kind of woman who didn't hesitate to strip naked and jump in my hot tub on our second or third date! My kind of gal!

Our relationship blossomed and soon she moved into my new home with me. A fan of clear and direct communication, I made it clear I wasn't looking for a roommate; I was looking for someone to share my home and start building a life together.

We did all the fun things in life that we enjoyed together. When she got home from work dinner would be cooking and a glass of wine would be waiting to help her transition from work to partner.

Having built National Legal Shield from the ground up I understood her business and we could spend time talking about her work when she needed to or wanted to. You see Elaine was and is a family law attorney.

Life as we were living it was good, we laughed, we loved, we talked, we traveled and we made plans together. So one day I asked Elaine to be my wife so that we could build our life together, us against the world. She said yes!

We were married in May of 1998 and honeymooned in Europe, with stops in Paris, Barcelona and then a cruise of the Mediterranean. Enjoying the French coast, Monte Carlo, a day trip into Rome, followed by stops in Sicily and Malta, what a grand trip.

But the honeymoon was short lived. Elaine seemed to be pulling away from me just a few months after our return. The physical closeness was no longer there and the intimacy had almost completely disappeared. What happened to that flirtatious, fun woman who so willingly jumped in my hot tub?

A few months after our wedding, Elaine told me that she was pregnant. Apparently she had known this for some time, but hadn't bothered to tell me. Her whole family had known for weeks, just not something she thought she needed to share with me. Elaine immediately moved out of the master bedroom into one of our guest bedrooms. She said that she was no longer comfortable sleeping in our waterbed. I offered to get a different bed. She said no that would not be necessary as she would move right back in after the baby was born.

I asked to join her in the spare bedroom but she said no she would be more comfortable sleeping alone while she was pregnant. Most evenings later in the pregnancy I would rub coconut butter on her belly to make her feel better and to help prevent stretch marks. I would read stories to Christopher while he was still "in the oven" and sing songs to him. Each evening, sooner or later Elaine would inform me that I had to leave the room.

I kept telling myself that it was just the pregnancy and the hormones and that things would get better after the baby was born. But I couldn't help wondering if the woman that I had met and fell in love with was gone for good.

I remember sitting in an appointment with Dr. Case, our OBGYN as she explained that it was good to have sexual intercourse to help near the end of the pregnancy. I had to quickly excuse myself from the office so that she would not see me cry. Intimacy in my life was over. Even though our doctor was recommending sex I knew that there was no way it was going to happen. My wife had cut me completely out of her life. She was all smiles to the outside world but when we were alone she made it perfectly clear that she no longer needed me or even wanted me.

After the birth of Christopher things got worse as opposed to better. I tried everything I could think of, counseling with our pastor, a marriage counselor, nothing helped. Finally one day out of desperation I wrote Elaine a letter. I asked her to "love me and be a real wife or let me go." I gave her the letter in which I had poured out my heart and waited for her reply, nothing. I waited three days, nothing, not a word.

So finally one night at the dinner table I said, "Elaine I gave you a letter three days ago and I was really hoping for a response." She said, "You want a response, here's your response… I'm going to take your money and your son, and I'm going to leave the state and you will never see him again."

I was devastated, I had hoped that the thought of our marriage ending would have caused her to recommit to our relationship. I filed for divorce and asked for joint custody. Elaine responded with a demand for sole custody. In Oregon the court can only order joint custody if both parents agree. All of the usual mediation and child custody evaluations were done and in the end the court awarded sole legal custody to me. I was so afraid of losing my son but it worked out as well as it could.

This is one of those catch 22's. I would like to say I wish I had never met her. Then I think of our son. If anyone came to me and said you can trade all of this for Christopher, it's a no brainer. Our son is the most precious gift. He makes all the bad memories bearable.

Chapter 12

Life can be wildly tragic at times, and I've had my share. But whatever happens to you, you have to keep a slightly comic attitude. In the final analysis, you have got not to forget to laugh.

~ *Katherine Hepburn*

Hindquarter of Beef

It was 1996 and another terrific 4th of July celebration. This one was being held at my Christmas tree farm outside of Dallas, Oregon. Fifty-one acres of noble fir and a handful of grand fir trees, most of them destined for the state of California once they matured. Teal Creek, which was more like a small river, ran through the middle of the property. There was a nice sandy beach for playing in the water, and we had developed a camping area where you could park an RV or camp trailer, or set up tents. We also had a sand volleyball pit. There was a regulation horseshoe setup, and a nice big fire ring.

I always had a good turnout for the 4th of July at my Christmas tree farm. Family, of course, along with neighbors and friends filled up our camp area. Tons of good food and the fireworks were imported from Wyoming . . . louder and much more spectacular than your normal home use fireworks. Everyone had fun singing along around the big fire pit well into the night. Few things feel better than waking up to the smell of eggs and bacon cooking over the fire, do you want pancakes with yours? On this particular 4th of July, that fire ring had a hindquarter of beef slowly roasting on a custom-made spit. What an amazing sight it was and mouth watering taste. Many of the people who attended that particular 4th of July celebration still talk about it today.

At sunset, everyone was around the campfire. They brought their guitars as usual. Everyone sang, we set off some fireworks, and had the obligatory s'mores for dessert, a great time. But the real story was that hindquarter of beef. That's what was different that year.

In the past, we had roasted turkeys, steak and chickens, but never a hindquarter of beef. It was kind of a surprise. It was actually a gift I received for giving some good advice. It started early one morning about six weeks before the 4th when my doorbell rang. It was my neighbor Nells. He and his wife Anne and their kids raised cattle and emus across the street from our Christmas tree farm. Nells said one of his steers had gotten loose and he wanted to know if he could come on my property and try to catch him. I said sure, and reminded him how much I liked to sleep in the morning. Next time, I told him, he didn't have to ask, he had my permission to just go catch his steer. So, Nells and his two boys Sven and Nells Gerhardt headed out across the field of trees trying to find their steer.

After about an hour, I'd had some coffee and breakfast and headed out to see how they were doing. They were still chasing that steer. He had gone across the river and up the bank, and was in the back field of trees. They were on foot hooting and hollering trying to herd that darn steer back toward their place. But this steer had no interest in getting caught. Nells needed help and so I offered to do whatever I could. We continued to try to herd the steer back toward their property, but every time he'd get where we thought he was headed in the right direction he would jump through a barbed wire fence into another field. Finally we concluded that we weren't going to persuade him to go back home just by hooting and hollering.

One of the boys thought they could lasso him, so he went and got his lariat. We spent the next hour and a half trying to lasso that steer. It was comical at first, but after two or three hours of chasing him, we were all getting kind of tired. I think Nells was getting a little more frustrated. They decided they were going to get their stock trailer.

By this time the steer was in the pasture of the neighbors north of my Christmas tree farm, so Nells asked their permission to go on the property, opened the gate, drove the stock trailer in there to set up some stock panels to create a funnel effect. He parked next to the fence and ran the panels out in a V from the other side of the trailer so we could herd the steer into the V and put an end to this nonsense.

Well, we finally got that steer up there and it looked like he was just about to go into the trailer when one of the boys shouted "Yahoo." That spooked the steer, and he turned and bolted back out, just about knocking Sven off his feet and off he went again.

Everybody was tired and frustrated by this point, and some of us were angry. I looked at Nells after having spent almost four hours trying to catch this animal and I told him if that steer was mine, I'd shoot him and be done with it. I told him I couldn't continue on as I had other things to do, and I headed back to my place.

About a week later there was a knock on the door. It was Nells again. He was kind enough this time to let me sleep in. "Hey," he said, "how would you like to have a hindquarter of beef for that 4th of July celebration you always do?" "That would be great," I said, "but what do you mean?"

He said, "Well, we kept trying to catch that steer and we never could, so I finally took your advice, went home and got my gun and put him down. Because of all your help and advice that finally resolved the problem, you can have a hindquarter for the BBQ if you want."

So that was the first time, and heck, the last time we ever had a hindquarter of beef for the 4th of July celebration. You talk about amazing, not only was it a sight watching that beef slow cooking over an open flame, but oh my goodness, that was the best beef I ever ate. And like I said, everybody still talks about it today.

What really matters in life are your personal relationships. I don't remember every deal I have ever done, but I will never forget that cow, the way it brought my neighbors, friends, family and I together, and the looks on everyone's face as they approached that fire pit with a fully-loaded spit turning for them. Kids and adults singing all night long and waking up to the smell of breakfast cooking over the fire. Not a year goes by that someone doesn't share with me about how much fun that year was for them as well.

Chapter 13

Happiness cannot be traveled to, owned, earned, worn or consumed. Happiness is the spiritual experience of living every minute with love, grace, and gratitude.

~ Denis Waitley

The Train Ride

The first trip that Christopher and I took alone together was after my divorce was final when he was about 5 ½ years old. It was a trip that both he and I remember fondly. We had reserved a sleeper car on an Amtrak Train headed south. The plan was to spend Christmas with my mother who lives in Eureka, California. The train was to depart the station in Salem, Oregon at three in the afternoon. It was about a 22-hour ride. I didn't realize how many stops a train could make and that the train was late getting out of the station, something I later learned is normal. When we finally boarded the train, the porter took our bags and showed us into our compartment.

It had a queen-size lower bunk for me and an upper bunk for Christopher. Our compartment had a nice big picture window for watching the scenery go by and its own private bathroom with a shower. If you reserve a sleeper car, you get priority seating for dining, so we made our way to the dining car at about six o'clock for dinner and had a delicious meal. I had expected the food to be somewhat akin to airline food. But it was actually a very good meal and to Christopher's and my surprise, we were treated to a hot fudge sundae for dessert.

After dinner we made our way back to the compartment, climbed onto the lower bunk together and got out the little portable DVD I had bought for the trip and watched a movie together. We talked and shared some stories when the movie was over and then Christopher climbed into his upper bunk, and we went to sleep to the rocking motion of the train. At about 1:30 in the morning I woke up, looked out that picture window and there was a beautiful sight… we were in the Siskiyou Mountains and there had been a fresh snowfall that day, the moon was full that night, and it was just aglow out. Our compartment was in a car three back from the engine and every time the train would go around a bend the strong headlights of the train would make the snow sparkle. I woke Christopher up and he came down on the lower bunk and we sat there curled up, him sitting in my lap facing out the window. It was an amazing sight. We just sat there silently, watching the trees go by all covered in snow. Then we drifted off back to sleep with that moon light streaming through our window. When we next awoke, Christopher said, "Dad, Dad! We are in California!! I know we are in California." And I asked, "How do you know," and he said, "Look… palm trees!" Sure enough there were some palm trees alongside the track.

Our train rolled into the Martinez station in the East Bay area of San Francisco, early in the morning, I don't remember it if was 7:00 a.m. or 9:00 a.m. but it was early. We were prepared to head on up to Eureka when we were told that we had to off load the train. I asked if we were switching to another train, and they told me, no there was no train service to Eureka and that you are going to have to go by bus. And I'm thinking, bus? We are supposed to be traveling first class, sleeper car all the way. The Amtrak folks insisted it was the end of the line for the train, so we gathered up all our stuff, got our bags from the porter and headed to the bus. We boarded for what was to be a ride far too long. About 11:00 at night the bus came to a stop right in the middle of the road. The rain was pouring down and everyone asked what was happening. The bus driver got on the microphone and said there had been a landslide and the highway was closed, we can't get to Eureka.

Mind you now, we have been traveling for hours and hours and hours on that bus. And we were about 40 miles from Eureka but there was no way to get through. The bus driver radioed his operations manager to see what he was to do and they told him to sit tight while they figured something out.

We sat there for about an hour on the bus. The bus driver talked to the Cal Trans people, the highway patrol, his operations manager, everyone was on the phone to everyone. They finally determined that not only was that slide area not going to be open that night, the highway would not be open again for at least a week. So they instructed the driver to turn around and head back down the highway to find a particular hotel. There were two young men on the bus who decided that since they were only 40 miles from Eureka and only 2 miles from the slide… they were going to call on their cell phones and have friends pick them up on the other side of the slide.

The bus driver told them they couldn't do that. Cal Trans told them they couldn't do that. But they said, OK we won't try to go through the slide but we are getting off the bus. Everyone knew full well they were going to try and sneak their way around. I have no idea what happened to those two young men. Hopefully they made it somewhere safe and sound because it was a stormy night and they were not prepared for the weather, and I doubt they had any concept of what a slide across the highway could look like. With Cal Trans and CHP at the site, there was no way they were going to get through, but nobody could convince them otherwise.

So we headed back down south on the windy highway, trying to find the hotel they had sent us to. The driver couldn't find the hotel so he pulled into a Burger King to ask for directions. The Burger King wasn't open, but there were a few employees in there cleaning up. While he was in there talking to the employees, two guys on the bus decided to commandeer the bus and they went up front, one jumped in the driver's seat and they started it up.

I was sitting up front and told them that regardless of how frustrated they were, that there was really no point in getting put in jail for grand theft auto, or bus in this case, and where did they think they were going to go? If you stay on the bus they are going to get us to a hotel and back to transportation that will get us all where we need to be. You don't want to steal the bus and if you are going to steal the bus, I want off and I bet a lot of other people do to. Everybody hollered them down and they got out of the driver's seat about the time the bus driver started running over when he heard the bus start up. Everybody was tired, everybody was cranky. Needless to say the bus driver was in a bad mood too. But he had gotten directions to the hotel and he got us there.

Since Christopher and I were sitting in the front, I could see the hotel as we pulled in and it wasn't that big. It wasn't really a hotel, it was a motel. I could see the cars in the parking lot and I could see they weren't going to have enough room for everybody. As soon as the bus stopped, I put Christopher on my shoulders as I bailed out the door and went directly to the office to make sure we could get a room. Turns out there really weren't enough rooms for everyone and the bus driver did not want to go somewhere else so the majority of the people had to sleep on the bus.

And no, the bus company did not pay for the rooms – that's why most of the people stayed on the bus, they didn't have the money for the room even if one had been available.

When we got up the next morning, they said that the highway going north was so badly damaged that it would take weeks and weeks to repair. There are no other north south routes to Eureka on the northern California coast. Their service did have one alternative, it would look like a giant triangle taking us away from our destination and then returning us. They would take us east all the way to Sacramento and then head back northwest on highway 299, a narrow and very crooked highway. With all of the scheduled stops and the out and back distance it would be a 14- hour ride! There was no other way to get to Eureka.

Christopher and I decided that really wasn't in the cards for us as much as we wanted to see Grandma Jinny. So we picked up the phone and called my buddy, Don. He and his wife Tina and their kids live just outside Santa Rosa, CA. I made arrangements for the bus driver to pull over on the side of the highway when we got to Santa Rosa and Don was waiting for us and we spent Christmas with Don's family.

One of the things that Christopher learned about on that trip was Hanukah. Tina was kind enough to do a little extra shopping and include Christopher in their Hanukah celebration, and he liked the idea of getting a new present everyday for 8 days. The stretched-out nature of the celebration seemed to beat the concept of Christmas for Christopher. He also learned about the miracle of the oil. We had a great time and when our time was up, we piled into Don's SUV and headed back to the train station at Martinez and rode the train back home. Thankfully, it was an uneventful ride home!

Chapter 14

*If you have love in your life, it can make up for a great many things
that are missing. If you don't have love in your life, no matter what
else there is, it's not enough.*

~ Ann Landers

How I Met my Wife and True Life Partner!

After helping edit the book time and time again, Carrie decided she wanted to tell a part of my story so here it is, in her words…

In early 2009, I guess the Universe had decided it had thrown enough crud at me (I'd been through a divorce and breast cancer in 2008) that it was time for something good to come my way. The delivery system? . . . eHarmony of course! Did I make it easy on the poor guy? Of course NOT! (stupid, stupid, stupid!) I made him work for it, but I knew from his profile, pictures and answers to my questions that he was special and someone I needed to get to know. So after three months of talking online, we set a date to meet. I almost cancelled, but somehow he knew and sent me the following email:

Don't lose your nerve girl… no matter what the future holds for us… something together or going our own separate ways… Thursday night will be a very fun evening, distracting us from the prying problems and challenges of life!

Looking forward to escaping from the world with you . . . David

How could I resist? He'd be the one in the cowboy boots he'd said. (That's the worst part about online dating you know… walking into a restaurant and trying to figure out which guy is the one you are supposed to meet.) I usually start with the face, but this time I was looking for the BOOTS! There's a pair…. Up, up, up my eyes went to find a 6'3" beaming, smiling, wonderful man who wrapped me in his arms to hug me hello, and I haven't left since!

Our first date lasted for hours as we talked and talked. I had explained to David, while drinking my glass of Oregon Pinot Noir, that the "Support Group" meeting I had been at that evening, and reason I could not meet him until late, was not AA, but a support group for women who had breast cancer. That's when I learned that he too, had been through cancer (much scarier then and still) than mine. This was just the first of many, many things we found we had in common and that form the solid foundation of our relationship. We both know how fragile life is and that what is most important is our love for each other and our family and friends. We know that "someday" may never come and that TODAY is someday and we make the best of each and every day we have together.

About a month after our first date, in the midst of a late spring snowstorm snuggled warm and tight in his cabin at the lake, David asked me to marry him. Of course I said yes, but it was still a little scary and happening all so fast. The Universe took care of all of that for me too… As we were driving home from the cabin, David turned on the radio in the truck. We were too far out of town still and there was so much static that he turned it off. Never to be deterred, he began to sing to me. We laughed and giggled our way down the road as he sang me silly love songs. His finale was "You Are the Woman That I Always Dreamed Of." His concert complete, and a few miles closer to town, he switched on the radio again. The first channel wasn't coming in clear so he switched to the next. Yep, you guessed it, THAT song was playing on the radio!! When was the last time you heard a Firefall song from the mid 70's?! I knew, right then and there that together, David and I and our boys were meant to be.

David's Story

After my divorce, but before I got sick, a friend of mine convinced me that I needed to date. He had great success with Match. com, and he was adamant that I needed to set up a profile. So with his help and wisdom we developed a profile on Match for me, uploaded some pictures and sure enough before long, I was dating.

I had a lot of fun, but what I found was that the majority of women just wanted to date. They were not interested in a serious relationship. I was looking for a partner, someone that I could go through life with, hand-in-hand. They could count on me and I could count on them.

Then I got sick and dating came to an end. As a matter of fact, when I came home from the doctor, I explained to the lady that I was dating that I had been diagnosed with cancer and she left. I mean left. Picked up her purse walked out of the house and I never saw her again. No phone calls, no e-mails, even though she was pushing me to marry her. My cancer diagnosis brought that to an end.

I put my shoulder to the grindstone and put my mind in the most positive place I could, and I marched forward, battling cancer. When my friends thought I'd gotten far enough down the road in my battle against cancer and that dating might be a good idea, they suggested Match.com again. But I wanted something better. I'd seen eHarmony's advertisements about real compatibility, so I decided that I was going to give that a try this time.

If you watch TV, you know that eHarmony has a patented algorithm with 29 levels of compatibility. It sounded like scientific mumbo-jumbo or advertising gobbledygook, but it became quickly apparent that the women eHarmony introduced me to were far superior from a relationship standpoint that I had ever seen from Match.com.

There was one profile, though, that stood out from all the rest. After seeing her picture and reading her profile I had a strong belief that Carrie was the one for me. I can't really explain it; it was just an overwhelming belief that we had to meet!

But Carrie's life did not seem settled, and I began to wonder if we would ever meet. After a few e-mails back and forth, but no date, Carrie explained that she was going on a family vacation for the holidays and would not be back until after the first of the year. So we agreed that we would get together upon her return.

The date for her return came and went, but no word from Carrie. Then I saw the update to her profile. She was back and had time to update her profile including some great photos from her trip to Fiji. But no contact with me, I knew that I would have to do something different to get her attention. So I sent this email to her:

Hi Carrie,

From the first time I read your profile something was different (must have been the "boot yoga" ha ha). I was/am drawn to you. I know that telling me what you did was not easy. But I want you to know how much it means to me that you were honest with me about it. It just confirms what I felt about you being different and someone I truly need to meet.

My birthday was Dec 6th... and we had a very fun and a very large party. Friends and family from all over the country came in, as well as the locals and we all had a great time! I cooked a Tapas feast and when it came time for the Champagne toast my 50 flutes were not enough to go around.

You get to choose what you are going to do and how you are going to handle it... but here is what I think. I think you should invest an hour of your time meeting me. If we hit it off, the way I think we will, it could help with your decision about your current situation. I am not asking you to go away on a trip or to make love with me... not even to join me for a fabulous dinner... just a glass of wine or a cup of coffee to see if we click.

Life is to short for regrets... you never know when your time will be up. So it is important to me to live a life without regrets... don't ever want to say, gee I wish I would have done this, or gee I wish I had done that. If we meet and hit it off, it would allow me the knowledge that I am actually waiting for something I know will be great. If we don't hit it off nobody has to wait for anything.

I will go with whatever you decide... if meeting for a glass of wine in some neutral out of the way place (so no one you know sees you) is just more that you can handle right now, I will just wait until you

are ready. But if you decide that life really is too short to sit around waiting for the good parts... then give me a call (or an email). No worries either way ;-)

Your friend... David

I knew in my heart that if we could meet we had a true chance at happiness. I could feel something was holding her back. I just did not know what it was. But my belief was so strong that I just could not give up. Well it worked, and Carrie finally agreed to meet for a glass of wine. Carrie made it clear that she would only have a little bit of time after a meeting just to squeeze in one glass of wine and a chance to talk.

I was standing in the entrance of the Dundee Bistro waiting for Carrie to arrive, and when she came through the door. Such a beautiful smile, I said to myself. "Oh #&%* I am toast." I just knew from that smile and warm hug that this was going to be as great as I had hoped.

I am happy to say we ended up closing that restaurant together, so many things to talk about, feeling so comfortable and so happy. Neither one of us wanted that evening to end, and we have been together ever since.

On May 24, 2009, just as we had envisioned . . . toes in the sand, warm breeze on our faces, and our boys by our side, we were married on McKenna Beach in Maui. *Yes that is the picture on the front cover.* The magic of our relationship seemed to follow us to the islands as the minister we spoke with over the phone could not have been more perfect in person. He remembered all that I had told him was important to us: family, respect, trust, and love; in his ceremony. When we exchanged rings, we also gave each of the boys a gold chain to wear as a symbol of our new family. They never take them off.

When Carrie and I got together, I shared with her what I knew about relationships and that the most important things were: honesty, trust and partnership. I explained to her that if she ever felt bad about something I said or something I did, then I was not communicating correctly. I told her, "All I ever want to do is to make you feel good and for you to be happy. If you are not happy, I am mis-communicating. Let me know right away and I will make adjustments and clear things up."

After our conversation, Carrie wrote in her journal… "What if there is never any ill intent behind anything either of us says or does?" "What kind of a relationship could we have?"

So, here we were on the same page once again; using our own individual words to express the same thing. We are partners, true partners and everything we do is to make our partner happy and to ensure that they know they are loved unconditionally every single day. Carrie asks herself this question every night… "By my words and actions today, does he KNOW that I am honored to be his wife?"

Recently, Carrie and I started working with a company called PAX. PAX is lead by Alison Armstrong, a warm and insightful woman who has spent 20 plus years studying the relationship between men and women. PAX's programs are centered around two important thoughts. First, "What if no-one is ever misbehaving?" Second, "What if there is always a good reason for everything our partners do?" Obviously our personal philosophy and that of PAX are a good match!

By studying and learning the reasons why men and women do and say what they do, and learning to acknowledge our differences, we are able to choose to work together in true partnership.

"WHAT IF NO ONE IS EVER MISBEHAVING?" WOW! What a thought!!!

You can access more information about Alison Armstrong and PAX via our website www.somedaygroup.com

Cancer

Chapter 15

We must be willing to get rid of the life we've planned, so as to have the life that is waiting for us. The old skin has to be shed before the new one can come.

~ Joseph Campbell

Cancer - It's a good thing I got it!

Who can say that about cancer? Well, in truth, there are several reasons I can.

First and foremost is the simple fact that I would not be here if not for the cancer diagnosis. The search for metastases led to the discovery of the massive pulmonary embolism. The filter that they placed in me caught it and literally saved my life!

Next... I never would have met Carrie. She and her two sons, Mitchel and Garret, along with my son, Christopher are now the foundations of happiness and meaning in my life, four pillars of joy and strength holding me up.

I was told to get my affairs in order. I did, I listened to what the doctors instructed, and I did it. Why was that a good thing? First, I sold all of my commercial and residential real estate before the crash in prices created by the mortgage mess. I was able to turn those holdings into liquid funds that I could live off of. So much better than landlord and management headaches that I would have been unable to deal with. Cash instead of tenants eliminated much of the stress in my life, letting me focus on Christopher and getting better. When God brought my new family, I was able to grab hold of them and live our new life together.

All of my retirement accounts and stock investments were liquidated into straight cash. Not a single equity product in my portfolio before the markets crashed. Thank you God, for looking out for me.

I am sure that the added stress of wondering where my next house payment would come from or even not knowing how I would put food on the table, that these added stresses could have pushed me over the edge.

We have all heard it said that stress kills. This is a situation where I know it's true. Even with the blessings I had, at times I could feel the stress pulling me into the deep, dark dungeon.

So if you are faced with this battle, or someone you know or love, someone you care about is faced with cancer, what can you do? What should you do? There are things that you can do that really help.

First, call them on the phone and just chat. Chat with them about anything, it does not have to be about the cancer. There is nothing to say about the cancer that will make it go away or make it better. Stop looking for the right thing to say. It just doesn't exist, acknowledge it, and then just let it go. Many times I saw that puzzled look on people's faces as they struggled to find the right thing to say. I always told them the same thing, don't worry, there are no perfect words, just let it go.

Tell your friends or loved ones who have cancer that you are sorry. Tell them that you are there to help, whatever they need--then tell them about how great your garden is doing. Once a week send a card or a note. Most people have no idea how moving human contact is; just a simple note will do – "Thinking of you." "Said a prayer for you today at church." "You will never guess what Joe did at the office today." Contact, simple human contact.

Drop by and clean the house, mow the lawn, or pull the weeds. Don't ask. If you can do it, just show up with supplies in hand. Make them a cup of tea and take them out to the garden with sunshine on their face and a blanket on their lap. You can just let them nap. Light some candles in the bathroom and draw them a bath.

Make a gift basket for the patient with a hat to keep their head warm, lip balm for those ever-dry lips, fragrance-free lotion, books to read, puzzles, and comfy cozy jammies. Or make a gift basket for the kids: games, books, videos, snacks, and toys to help keep them occupied during doctor appointments or hospital visits.

You can take the kids off their hands for an afternoon or overnight. One popular activity for the ladies is a wig party -- it makes the transition easier and it is loads of fun for everyone. Remember that laughter is the best medicine.

Deliver dinners ready to go, it will mean far more than you can imagine. Get them a gift certificate for their favorite restaurant if they feel well enough to eat and strong enough to go out. They can dine in, if not, "to go" is always a great option.

It is very hard for most people to ask for and accept help. Do it anyway; read between the lines to find out what they need most. Little things mean just as much as big things. It says you care and are thinking about them. They get to remember, by every act no matter how large or small, that they are blessed.

It's sad that money is such a big part of life now, with most of the world feeling lucky if they can just live paycheck to paycheck. Every little bit will help. You don't have to rely on your own pocket. Put out those collection jars for change, any kind of fundraiser, no matter how large or small, will be greatly appreciated. Carrie and I got together with friends and helped to put together a benefit concert to raise funds for a dear friend of ours. It was a great success and the show was fun, and we even did an auction during the show. Be creative, have fun. Give everyone a chance to show that they care.

If you are the one who is sick, you need to relax and learn how to receive and accept the help offered, it's done out of love. So what if the house isn't clean to your standards – let it go! So what if the laundry isn't folded the way you do it – let it go! Think about what you would do for your friend and be a good friend in return – let your friends take care of you this time.

I have received the greatest gift of all . . . time. More time to raise Christopher. Plus now I get to share those same life lessons with Mitchel and Garret as well.

So as I told you, it truly is a good thing I got Cancer. For these reasons and so many more, every day as my life continues on - one joyful discovery after another.

Thank you God!

Chapter 16

If you woke up this morning with more health than illness, you are more blessed than the million who will not survive the week.

If you have food in your refrigerator, clothes on your back, a roof over your head and a place to sleep, you are richer than 75 percent of the world.

If you have money in the bank or in your wallet, you are among the top 80 percent of the worlds wealthy.

If you hold up your head with a smile on your face and are truly thankful, you are blessed because the majority can, but most do not.

~ Author Unknown

The Basic Plan for Kicking Cancer's Butt

When the first MRI confirmed that I had some sort of tumor growing on the base of my spine, my family doctor, Michael Kelber, referred me to Dr. Pierce. Dr. Pierce is an oncologist who practices at the Hematology and Oncology Center at the Salem Hospital. He is an excellent doctor who can talk faster than any other human being that I have ever met. It is important to take written notes with you to your doctor appointments or he will be done and gone before you can remember what to ask. He is helped by a team in the office but my main contact was with Kelly. She was so very helpful and caring making the whole process easier to go through.

Before I knew it, I had three teams of doctors working to figure out what was wrong with me and how they would go about trying to save my life. The head of the cancer unit at Oregon Health & Science University (OHSU) that specialized in my type of cancer was Dr. Ryan. I met with Dr. Ryan and his team; they did lots of poking and prodding. And then they referred me to the orthopedic surgical unit for oncology, where I was assigned to Dr. Krajbich. His team took their turn, poking and prodding.

Each of these three groups of doctors and their staff (Dr. Pierce in Salem, Dr. Ryan, and Dr. Krajbich and their teams up at OHSU) worked in unison in an attempt to diagnose the type of cancer I had and to formulate a plan for treating the cancer. Even though they did not have an exact diagnosis yet, it was decided that my treatment would begin with three rounds of chemotherapy. Then Dr. Krajbich and his team would do surgery to remove what they could of the tumor. Once I recovered from that surgery, the plan was for three more rounds of chemotherapy.

The initial plan was for all treatment to be done at OHSU. When I spoke with Dr. Pierce about the possibility of receiving my chemotherapy in the Salem Hospital, he indicated that that would be fine, and so that is the decision I made. There were two reasons for this decision. The first one was I felt most comfortable with Dr. Pierce. The second factor was I had been Mr. Mom since the day Christopher was born and the thought of spending an extended amount of time in a hospital in Portland where he would not be able to come and see me, would simply not work for me. Little did I know how difficult it would be for Christopher to see me regardless of where I had my chemo.

I had never been around cancer. No friends, no family members had ever had cancer. This was all new to me. The extent of my knowledge going into this was what I had seen in movies and while watching some tear-jerking movie of the week on TV. They all portray it as a very bad experience that most people did not survive. I have always tried to keep up with the news so I was aware that the survival rates for cancer were improving across the board.

I learned that not only are there many different types of cancer, there are many different varieties of chemotherapy drugs. Most of the improvements in the survival rate were coming from two areas; early detection and targeted chemo drugs. Nope, we did not catch mine early. It was rather large in size and had grown through my coccyx bone and tangled itself around the base of my spine in the nerve tree area.

As for those targeted chemo drugs, the ones that can magically focus on just your cancer cells and not kill every other living cell in your body, nope, not for me. No targeted chemo drug has been developed for my kind of cancer, so I am stuck with the two oldest and most destructive chemo drugs, Adriamycin and Cisplatin.

One of them is called "Big Red" because the solution in the IV bag is very red in color; you can see it from across the room as it hangs on the IV stand and slowly drips into your body. My chemotherapy would have to be administered on an inpatient basis, and I would be there for several days. The targeted chemotherapy patients can be out the same day after just a few hours.

Life became a whirlwind of tests, doctor appointments, and making arrangements for Christopher's care. I had a lot to learn, most of which I wish I didn't ever learn. Chemo, here I come!

Chapter 17

Uncertainly is the refuge of hope.

~ Henri Frederic Amiel

Diagnosis, What Diagnosis?

Once you get that initial diagnosis of cancer, the doctors need to determine several things. Has it spread? What kind of cancer is it? The answer to each of these questions will have a major impact on your treatment plan.

In my case a series of procedures were done to help find the answers. They started with a whole body bone scan on the 3rd of March using an MRI machine. Then on March 7th a CT scan was done in a two-step process. First they did a CT of my chest, abdomen, and pelvis area. Then a contrast dye was injected and the CT scans were done again for each of those areas. Two things were found, the first was a very large destructive mass, which was listed as most likely "chordoma" (an especially nasty form of cancer). The second thing they found was a massive pulmonary embolism. I needed a filter placed in my vena cava (the main vein from the lungs to the heart) immediately or I could die.

I was under the knife on the 9th of March so that the filter could be implanted to hopefully catch the embolism if it broke loose. As part of my cancer treatment plan, a CT-guided needle biopsy into the bone at the base of my spine was also planned for the same day. The purpose of the biopsy was to confirm the diagnosis of chordoma.

The surgical procedure was to start with me on my back and place the filter. Once the filter was in place and the fear of an embolism reaching my heart and killing me was reduced, they would roll me over and do the biopsy deep into the base of my spine. With the help of general anesthesia I went to sleep on my back expecting to wake up in the recovery room sometime later in the same position.

It did not quite work out that way. I came to on my stomach with a feeling of intense pain in my lower back. I heard a noise and felt an impact in my lower back area. I looked back over my shoulder and saw a doctor raising his hand with some sort of mallet in it ready to swing at me. I asked, "Is this supposed to hurt this much?" The Doctor stopped mid swing and I heard these words, *"HE'S TALKING!"* I can only guess that someone made the proper adjustment to my anesthesia because I don't remember anything else until I awoke in recovery. But I will never forget that pain, that pressure, or those words, *"HE'S TALKING!"* The surgeon was using the mallet to "tap" a 13-guage bone biopsy needle into place. For non-medical folks, that's a really big needle. Now I just had to wait for the results.

Everyone I have talked with who has gone through things like this, has shared that the waiting is the hardest part. There's no choice in the matter but waiting encourages your mind to run free, usually in a negative direction. Lucky for me I did not have to wait too long for the results of my biopsy. But I thought that biopsy results would mean a diagnosis. I was not aware that I would have to wait a very long time for a true, solid diagnosis.

The results of this biopsy were given to my Oncologist, Dr Pierce, on the 10th of March. The result stated, "There were no diagnostic abnormalities." I had gone through the process and the pain, even got to wake up in the middle of it all for a diagnosis of "NO Diagnosis." Still waiting, still wondering, is it chordoma? Can it be treated or am I really going to die and leave my son without a father? I had waited so long for Christopher to come along. Yet here I am wondering if I am going to be here to raise him.

Doctor Pierce said that he was suspicious about the test results and that he was going to send me up to OHSU, Oregon Health & Science University, the premier medical facility in the Northwest. Dr. Pierce's notes stated "I do not favor additional biopsy attempts in Salem." I later learned that the Doctor who did the biopsy in Salem decided that he was so good at it, and that, despite the medical order by my Oncologist for a CT guided biopsy, he could do the job without using the CT that was right there to guide the needle. Hey, people fly blind and it works out sometimes, right?

With a new CT guided biopsy ordered at OHSU, it was time to meet the Doppler machine. You have heard of his cousin on the news during the weather report. They use Doppler radar to determine the weather. In my case they used the Doppler machine to determine whether or not I had any additional blood clots or if the oral medicine (Coumadin) that I was taking was working on the pulmonary embolism that they had found earlier. Coumadin is actually a rat poison that they somehow discovered thins your blood. If they give it to you in the correct amounts, it can cause a clot to disintegrate. It also helps to prevent the formation of any new clots. But you have to endure constant blood draws to check your clotting factor. My medic alert bracelet lets people know that I am on Coumadin just in case I can't speak for myself.

On March 16th I entered the Salem hospital and underwent the Doppler study. The result read "abnormal with a nonoclusive clot on right side." The next day I had yet another "enhanced chest CT" (that means with contrast dye injected into my bloodstream). I got the results of this test right away and it stated, "The pulmonary embolus in the lower right lobe appears smaller than it was on 3-7-06." The Coumadin that I was taking to thin my blood and eliminate the clot was starting to do its job.

The filter put in place to catch the embolism could only stay in for a maximum of about 14 days. After that it can become impossible to remove because the tissue starts to grow around those barbs holding it into place. So on the 21st of March I was admitted to the Salem hospital for the removal of the filter. Taking it out is kind of a cool procedure (as long as you don't think about the fact that they are fishing in your jugular).

The surgeon makes an incision in the jugular vein on your neck and inserts a guide wire sleeve along all the way down the vein until it reaches the spot where the filter is. On the leading edge of the filter is a small islet. The surgeon can advance the interior wire, which has a hook on the end of it, from the sleeve as he attempts to hook the islet on the end of the filter. If they are unable to hook that islet, the filter stays. When they do hook the islet, sometimes the filter still can't be removed from the vein because it has grown into the tissue too much and won't come loose; then it has to stay. If the filter must remain, your body requires blood thinners for the rest of your life. This makes simple falls or even a minor car accident, a serious concern. While you are on blood thinners, your body cannot clot its blood normally, so you have to be watched very closely. I am happy to report that my surgeon is an excellent fishermen and my filter was removed without any trouble whatsoever.

Being on blood thinners impacts my life on a daily basis. I have to go into the hospital regularly, once every week or two, to have my blood checked for its clotting factor. The INR clotting factor is a careful balance that is affected not only by the drugs but is also affected by food choices, alcohol, wine, exercise, and most other day-to-day medicines. Every new medication that goes into my body must be cleared with the anticoagulation clinic.

When I have medical procedures that could involve bleeding, the doctors must "build a bridge" with a fast-acting anticoagulant. These are great fun! I get to self inject them subcutaneously (under the skin), a good sized needle into my stomach twice a day for a week or two before and after just to go to the dentist. As well as any other procedures that will or might cause bleeding. It burns going in and looks great too, like someone hit you repeatedly across the stomach with a baseball bat, massive ugly bruises running across your stomach.

Before the next biopsy was performed, I was told not to get my hopes up, but there was a slight chance that it might not be chordoma after all. Dr Krajbich said that even though everything seemed to point to chordoma, he had never seen it hide this way. If it truly was chordoma we should have had a diagnosis by now. There was a one in a million chance that it's not chordoma after all!

On the 24th of March another needle biopsy was done, this time with the help of the CT for guidance. It was done in Portland at OHSU per my Oncologist's request. Unfortunately the result was the same – inconclusive! This really sucked, I mean really. It is so hard to just keep waiting, not knowing.

All the doctors have been saying the same thing, chordoma. Looks like chordoma, acts like chordoma. I learned the hard way when they tell you that it's chordoma don't, under any circumstances, go to your computer and Google "chordoma." You talk about ugly… if there was hope living somewhere deep down inside you, those search results can stamp it right out. Work with your doctors and wait to get a diagnosis first so that you're not worrying about conditions you might not even have. Google or some stranger at the coffee shop (trust me they are happy to interject their opinion) have no true idea about your condition, so wait for the diagnosis.

When it came to sharing everything that was happening to me, on a day-to-day basis, I was not that good at it. Communicating was very difficult, everyone who knew me and cared about me wanted to know how I was. Are you OK? Are the treatments helping you? Is the chemotherapy as bad as they say? All fair questions and I wanted to answer them. It just became more and more painful each time I had to repeat what seemed to be a never-ending litany of bad news. I was surviving by keeping my sense of humor, by staying positive as best I could.

Repeating the same negative crap over and over again made staying positive, nearly impossible. So I created an email group. Wow, what a simple idea, but one that let me share with all of the people in my life. Sharing without dragging myself deeper and deeper down into despair with each phone call became impossible. (If someone in your life is in my situation, please share this idea with them… I hope it helps).

Here is the email that I sent out to my cancer group after my conversation with Doctor Krajbich:

-----Original Message-----
From: David Koop
Sent: Friday, March 24, 2006 8:50 AM
To: DAK (E-mail)
Subject: DAK - update

So I met with DR. Krajbich at OHSU. He too believes that it is Chordoma. There is a one in a million chance that it might not be. Because of the severe consequences of the surgery and treatment for Chordoma he wants to be absolutely positive. So today at 3pm I will be checking into the OHSU hospital for a surgical biopsy under general anesthesia. They will be cutting out a piece after seeing it with their own eyes so as not to come up with a miss like last time. The sample will be sent to pathology while I am still under to confirm that it is the sample they need. They will then sew me back up and keep me overnight.

It takes about five days to get the results.

Thank You for all of your prayers and good wishes . . .I love you all . . .

David

PS: OHSU is Oregon Health Sciences University

Several times from several sources during the first few months I heard, "Get your affairs in order." Not only is your life over, it is going to be a horrible end. So I listened to what they said, and I got my affairs in order. I sold all of my businesses. I cashed out all of my investments, and I sold all of my real estate holdings that I could.

I have been very lucky in my life and have done well enough that I could focus on spending what time I had left with my son and focus on fighting the cancer. It has been and continues to be a very difficult fight. But I cannot imagine trying to do that and worry about putting food on the table or wondering where the next house payment would come from. The added stress would have been unbearable. So I thanked God for the blessings that I had and I pushed on.

I showed up at OHSU for yet another biopsy… what would we find this time? Seven days later everyone in my cancer email group got the news in the following email.

-----Original Message-----

From: David Koop
Sent: Friday, March 31, 2006 11:52 AM
To: DAK (E-mail)

Holy S*&%, oh my GOD

You know that 1 chance in a 1,000,000 . . .well it turns out that I am the LUCKIEST man in the world!!!!

Not only did the body scans to detect the spread of the cancer find a pulmonary embolism that would have killed me on the spot, got that under control.

The open surgical biopsy came back NEGATIVE for Chordoma, NOT cancer at all!!!

The power of all your prayers and good thoughts . . .Thank You all. I am now back to the beginning, what is it and how are we going to fix it. But it is NOT cancer.

I love and care for each and every one of you sooooo much and I hope you know that I felt and appreciated all of your good energy, thoughts, love and prayers.

Christopher's Dad Alive and well for a long time to come!!!

Talk about a one in a million chance, I finally got the call I had been waiting for. Not only was it not chordoma... but, they said it was "NOT EVEN CANCER!"

I can't tell you how that felt... not even cancer... OMG!!! I quickly shared the good news with all of my friends and family. I don't know of a time when I was happier or a time where I could actually feel the weight lifted off my shoulders . . . NOT EVEN CANCER???

All the things I was worried that I would miss out on, now I can do them all and more. I could go back to a normal life without all of this disease and treatments to worry about. No more stress wondering if it is chordoma or if it is some other kind of cancer, has it spread, will it spread? Raising Christopher, traveling, building yet another business if I wanted to – I could start to live again! Yes! Time with Christopher, thank you God.

Then five hours later the call that dropped like a ton of bricks. I am not even sure of his exact words, but here is the gist. Dr. Krajbich said he was sorry, so very sorry; I should never have received the phone call about not having cancer. "That information was wrong. It **IS** cancer and we need to get in there right away and remove everything that is left."

-----Original Message-----
From: David Koop
Sent: Friday, March 31, 2006 4:47 PM
To: DAK (E-mail)
Subject:

Well . . . welcome to my world.

The roller coaster continues.

I just got off the phone with Doctor Krajbich. The orthopedic oncologist who did the biopsy. When someone else told me this morning that the test was negative...I asked what that meant, they said "You do not have cancer."

Doctor Krajbich said "not the case"... just did not have as good of a sample as they thought and needed. The pathologist told him that they thought they had some Chordoma cells but could not be sure because of the large number of reactive cells.

Bottom line is they are scheduling me for yet another biopsy early next week.

I am sooooo sorry to have taken all of you on this ride with me. I guess roller coasters really can make you sick some times.

Start praying again (and if anyone is listening to your prayers let them know my sense of humor is all gone).

David

Here is the cancer group email that went out while waiting to get the approval from insurance, even the insurance company had a hard time believing that we still did not have a diagnosis.

-----Original Message-----
From: David Koop
To: DAK (E-mail)
Sent: Fri, 7 Apr 2006 16:03:08 -0700

Hi everybody!

Well it is Friday and the 3rd biopsy that was to be performed the first part of this week has not happened. First couple of times I heard that the insurance would not approve it... don't know what is up now. Yes I have left several messages and am waiting by the phone like a little school girl hoping for a date.

Got a call from OHSU scheduling a few days ago... seems as though my real deal surgery is set for April 19th. Yeah I know they have not completed my latest biopsy but they have scheduled my surgery???

Dr. Krajbich is out of the country until the 17th. So I called my oncologist here in Salem, Dr. Pierce to talk with him about what is going on and what he thinks about it.. guess what he is also out of the country until the 17th... noooo there is not an oncologist convention at some remote locale, he is in Rome with his wife, travel and return dates are just a coincidence... just leaves me with no one to talk to until the 17th.

When I called Amy, Dr. Krajbich's medical assistant to ask about the scheduled surgery she said that the doctor had requested it but that she did not know when they would be doing the reconstructive surgery...silly me I did not even know I was going to be needing reconstruction. Seems that I always have something new or more to look forward to???

Oh yeah... almost forgot... the incision in my backside is infected... they are treating it with antibiotics. Staples are sooooo much fun.

Because of all the fun listed above and a dramatic rise in the pain level this has been a fairly tuff and depressing week, but we are to have sunshine this weekend... maybe I can work on the income taxes outside on the deck...standing up of course.

I will let you know more when I know more... Thank You for all the prayers and warm thoughts... David

On April 13th of 2006, a needle biopsy was done at OHSU. It was CT guided but the results were "non – diagnostic." How hard can this be how much do I have to go through? This is the THIRD time a biopsy has been performed and they still can't tell me IF its cancer let alone what kind it is? Are you kidding me?

Here is the next cancer group email:

Date: Thu, 13 Apr 2006 23:49:18 -0700
From: David Koop
To: DAK (E-Mail)
Subject:
Well biopsy number three is in the books.

It was to take just under one hour to complete but as we have all learned I just don't do things the easy way. They had a little trouble getting what they needed. Everyone was aware of how important getting an accurate diagnosis is this time and the problems we had in the past, soooo after about the first hour they called down the pathologist who worked with the team to make sure they got what they needed. It took them three hours but.....

This procedure was a CT guided biopsy. They took many samples from several areas. After a lot of work they all believe that they got some very good samples in the end (no pun intended). They are extremely confident that the will be able to get a clear diagnosis. I hope they are right.

I brought to their attention the problem of my waking up in the middle of the first biopsy, soooo they came up with a guaranteed way to ensure that it would not happen this time... conscious sedation... that's right I got to be awake for the whole thing!!!

As you all know I am scheduled for surgery on the 19th. They say it will take about six hours to complete if all goes well. The results of this biopsy will help to guide them as to how much of me they have to remove.

Sorry for no phone calls today but I just wasn't up for it.

I need all of your prayers, your good thoughts and your support as I go into this next phase. You have all helped to carry me this far and I love each and every one of you. My life has been so special because of the times we have had together. It is comforting to me to know that you all are there for me. It is difficult to explain in words how as it gets darker in my thoughts that each of you in some way brings in light and hope... Thank You!

Tonight I would ask that you also give a special prayer for Christopher. You all know how much he means to me, and he is worried about his dad. Impossible to hide the fact that I keep ending up at the hospital.

Well time for some more pain meds and some sleep. Good night...David

My doctors were as fed up as I was with the lack of a diagnosis after three needle biopsies and on April 19th a team of surgeons at OHSU preformed the final biopsy. This time they did away with the needles and the mallets and performed an open surgical biopsy. Their goal was to remove as much of the tumor as possible. I got to stay awake for this one too, lucky me. I was put into a state of sedated consciousness and they opened me up like a Thanksgiving turkey. Once I was open they reached for a Rongeurs, it's a tool that the doctor used like an ice cream scoop to dig into and remove everything inside the bone, the tumor, marrow, bone fragments and anything else that got in the way. The official name of the procedure: Excisional Biopsy of the Sacrum with Bone Grafting.

This procedure was full of possible complications because they were working through and around my spinal cord and all of the nerves that branch out at the base of the spine. Death, blindness, paralysis, incontinence, colostomy bag, and impotence were prominent on the consent form I had to sign.

The procedure was so invasive and traumatic that I could only be discharged after three days in the hospital. I was only then allowed to go home because of the promise of 24-hour care.

Date: Tue, 25 Apr 2006 00:22:23 -0700
From: David Koop
To: DAK (E-mail)
Subject:

Just a quick update until the meds kick in.

Before the surgery on Wed we got the path report back.. You know third time is a charm... no such luck. No diagnosis again. So instead of doing the Chordoma surgery with its horrible results, or doing another biopsy expecting a different result... they did the following.

The entire tumor was removed, but not the sacrum and all the surrounding tissues...so much for the half assed jokes I was working on. The list of consequences had the same items on it for this surgery, but the chances for those bad results were much less.

When I woke up in recovery I was happy to see that I had not lost my vision, I then looked at my toes and wiggled them, yes they moved!!! Then I ran my hand up my left side and down my right side... no colostomy bag... seems like a good result to me.

At some point maybe I will tell you about the drug change... very bad idea.

I was released from OHSU on Fri at 11:30 am

By 1:30pm on Sat I was in the emergency room at Salem Hospital. I had severe chest pains, difficulty breathing, and sick to my stomach. The on call doctor at OHSU said get to the Emergency room immediately. They had me chew 4 aspirin (not designed with taste or chewing in mind) then hooked me up to the EKG machine and got a abnormal EKG report. They put one then another Nitro pill under my tongue. Then they hung an IV of nitro.

I was taken to the CT lab for a contrast spiral CT. No new clots even thought they could not seem to get me back on the fragmin at the hospital, more on that another time.

Tests for blood gasses were done, two were ok one came back as abnormal (we know him!) I was held overnight because the blood gas test doesn't report accurately until more than 6 to 8 hours after the event.

The blood gas test overnight and in the morning came back the same as the first one. It was decided that the abnormal report was most likely caused by the surgery.
I was discharged from Salem Hospital about 12 noon.

I still know the same things I did before... Is it Chordoma... They don't know. What happened Sat... They don't know.

There is some sort of condition or something... I forget the name that mimics a heart attack... maybe that was it... Who knows? They want to do more tests, like a stress test, but my body is in no condition at this time. So once again we shall wait.

As for the other I await the path results, since they have the whole damn thing it will be impossible to say we don't have a good sample... I have no more samples to give.

On the good news front the surgeon says he has never seen Chordoma hide like this before and he is hopeful for a good result.

Good night... Love you all... David

"No result, no result and no result" had been my only answer while trying to find a diagnosis. But this was the one, the final biopsy. Hey they opened me up, all the way open and took it out, the entire tumor (that they could see) was removed. Surely we would know now what we were dealing with.

All of that and we still didn't have a diagnosis! Biopsy after biopsy, different hospitals, different doctors, with CT guidance, without CT guidance and still no definitive diagnosis? The last one that opened me up all the way surgically and then scooped out the entire tumor. They have the whole thing to look at and we are still not sure?

Well it was getting harder and harder to keep my sense of humor about all of this.

Finally – a diagnosis!

Date: Wed, 3 May 2006 14:03:48 -0700
From: David Koop
To: DAK (E-Mail)
Subject:

Soooooooooo here we go.

Good news... it is not Chordoma

Bad news... it is Osteo Sarcoma

Good news... this one responds to chemo

Bad news... the new chemo drugs that target only the cancer don't work on this one

Good news... it is not chordoma

Bad news... this one is way, way more aggressive

Good news... they hope to start chemo on tue (if they can get the insurance on board)

Bad news... it is the old chemo drugs that do havoc to your whole body

They plan for me to be in the hospital for three days if all goes well, then home avoiding any and all sick people since my immune system will be suppressed. three weeks later all over again. Then tree weeks later for a third time. At that time they will do the wide resection surgery.

If there are no live cancer cells in what they take out, they will do another three rounds of chemo... if there are live cells they will have to re evaluate the next course.

This normally attacks teenage boys in the knee. Unfortunately the success rate in people my age is not anywhere as good.

BUT with this one I do have a chance !!!

Love you all... please keep up the prayers for me and Christopher... David

Chapter 18

When life gives you a hundred reasons to cry, show life that you have a thousand reasons to smile.

~ Author Unknown

Round One:
I Lost It!

Through my whole ordeal with Cancer, I only lost self control one time.

I was getting ready for the first round of chemotherapy with those non-targeted drugs. I remember hearing stories and seeing representations in movies about how bad chemotherapy is. So it's very difficult to freely decide to get up in the morning, get into the car, go to the hospital and then check-in voluntarily, knowing full well what the doctor's plan is for you.

Luckily I had my friend, Tito, who came up to help me. Tito and his wife Kathy live in Oxnard, California. We have known each other through business for about 16 years, and have been very close friends for about a decade. Kathy was kind enough to loan me her husband. I know because of our bond that Tito will always be there for me if I truly need him, but it was nice that Kathy was onboard too. I have three best friends, people that I know that I can reach out to when I need them and they will be there.

Tito kept talking to me all morning as we got ready and during the drive over to the hospital. We sat in the waiting area together and then went up to the desk to check in when my name was called. They assigned me a room on what they affectionately call "Five South." I soon learned that is where all us cancer patients hang out.

With my room assignment in hand, we went to the elevator and the young lady at the reception area escorted us down the hall on the fifth floor until we got to my room. It was a private room with a decent view of the trees and some of the other hospital buildings across the street.

For the next hour or so we mostly just sat and talked. Nurses came in and out, weighed me and measured how tall I was. I could tell Tito was getting a little antsy. He didn't seem comfortable there in the hospital. He kept asking if there was anything that I might want. "Do you want me to go get you anything?" "You need a hamburger?" "You want me to go get you a mocha?"

Tito was like a caged animal -- not happy, pacing back and forth, back and forth. Finally he said, "Okay big guy, I'm going to go, I'll come back later." And with that I was alone in my room.

At long last the nurses came in and gave me the hospital gown that they wanted me to change into and said I needed to get into bed. Now mind you I had arrived at the hospital at 7:00 a.m. and it's now about 9:00 a.m. I do as they ask and put on my gown and get in bed. Tito is long gone and I'm twiddling my thumbs. I turn on the TV and watch some cooking shows just killing time. Finally, I buzzed the nurse. When she came into the room I asked, "Hey what's the deal?"

She said that the prescription for my chemo drugs had to be called into the pharmacy downstairs, the order had to be filled and then when it was ready they would buzz us. "Then I will bring it up and get you started," she said. I asked how much longer? She replied that it would still be quite a while yet.

For the rest of the day I laid in bed twiddling my thumbs. Finally I watched a few more cooking shows and caught up on the news. All day long, three different nurses were coming in and out of the room, and I was my being my normal gregarious self, laughing, joking and having a good time trying not to let the wait get to me.

Finally, I asked the nurse, "Hey, when are we going to get this show on the road? It's four o'clock in the afternoon and I'm still waiting. Why did I have to be there at six or seven in the morning and then just wait and wait all day? Is this normal?" "Oh no, oh no it's not normal," she said.

Finally, about five thirty or six o'clock in the evening a nurse came into the room and shared the good news that my chemo drug prescription had been filled and they could bring it up.

I waited and waited and waited for those magical chemo drugs to appear. And I waited and I waited about an hour before I finally heard the door open. I looked to my left and coming into the room were two people in complete hazardous material suits. I'm talking the gowns, the gloves, the masks. I couldn't believe it. I thought it was a joke. Seriously, I thought it was a joke. I'd been laughing and joking with them all day and I thought they were joking back.

But they were not joking. They said, "No, with these chemo drugs that you're taking we have to wear these HAZMAT suits." It was startling, it was frightening. "Get out!" I said, and they looked at me kind of strange thinking I'm joking again. "Get the f*ck out of my room now!" I yelled. I was not joking. I was freaking out. I was losing it.

I couldn't believe that this stuff was so dangerous that they had to wear a full hazardous materials suit just to carry it. "If this stuff is so dangerous that you have to wear a full HAZMAT suit just to carry it, there's no f*cking way you're putting it in my body. Get out! Get out of my room! You're not putting that f*cking stuff in my body."

After awhile, one of the nurses came back into the room and asked if I was okay. I asked him "Why, why do you have to wear the suits? Why would you show up in full gear without telling me ahead of time? If you care about your patients, don't ever blindside anyone like that again. Give them fair warning, help them understand what to expect, help them understand what's coming. Show a little compassion, help your patients. This is difficult enough as it is without this kind of horrifying surprise." I could see the pain on their faces. They could see that in their efforts to make me feel better, to get me better they had done just the opposite. I am sure that no one else in the future will get the surprise that I did.

So yeah I lost it, I mean I completely lost control. It was the first time and the only time during the process. But the way they did it was uncalled for, it wasn't necessary, and I certainly hope that they learned from my experience to be more compassionate with their patients in the future.

I don't want to give you the wrong impression, though. During my experience with this cancer and my cancer treatments I was treated in two different facilities. For the original biopsy and the actual rounds of chemo I was treated at Salem Hospital. For all of the other biopsies and the open surgical biopsies as well as the major surgery to remove the base of my spine, I was treated at the Oregon Science and Health University (OHSU). They are an internationally renowned group of caregivers.

The level of expertise that they provide is unsurpassed anywhere in the world. I'm not supposed to be walking and I am. The medical consensuses was that, following surgery, I would be paralyzed from the waist down and have a colostomy bag to deal with as well.

Dr. Krajbich, my surgeon, is the most amazing fellow and a miracle worker to boot. When I Googled him, I saw posting after posting from patients and parents of children who have been treated as a last resort by Ivan. Time after time he's been able to work miracles where everyone else had felt there was no hope.

The surgery to remove the base of my spine was extremely difficult because that's where the nerve tree is. That's the branching out of nerves from the spinal cord at its base. I have no idea how these surgeons can do this, I'm only thankful that they can.

So yes, I was taken aback by the HAZMAT suits, but the level of care that I was given at Salem Hospital from a loving, nurturing "Let's make the patient feel as comfortable as possible perspective" was far above that at OHSU, where they were cold and clinical.

One of the best examples I can give was during my first round of chemo at Salem Hospital. One of my nurses came into my room. I had just finished a horrible and extended round of vomiting. I was sitting on the edge of my bed feeling like death warmed over or perhaps that death would even be preferable at that point. It's hard to explain, when it just won't quit and you feel like you can't breathe. You just can't catch your breath and you feel like you are suffocating.

I guess she could just see it in my eyes or my face but she knew. She just knew that I needed a hug. Just a simple hug, but at that moment it meant the world to me! She stepped up to the edge of the bed where I was sitting. She just held me, not saying a word. Just holding me and gently rubbing her hands up and down my back. Then after a few minutes she said "You poor dear, I have worked here for over 23 years and I have never seen anyone as sick as you."

Hey, I learned a new word though! "Emesis." Yeah in addition to just plain old nausea, I am suffering from Emesis. Commonly known as delayed vomiting. They tell me it normally occurs two to five days after they start the Cisplatin. Emesis is different from acute vomiting because it is particularly difficult to control with standard drugs.

I had to deal with a lot of things while lying in that hospital bed. I had a lot of thoughts going through my mind. I will tell you the most difficult thing for me was laying in the hospital bed watching the chemotherapy drugs slowly drip, drip and drip into my ever weakening body, knowing Christopher was just 10 minutes away and that I could not see him.

Since he was born I had been Mr. Mom. Hey, I was the first man to be active in the West Salem Mothers Club! My business was set up so that I could spend most of my time raising my son. I had waited my whole life for him to come along, and I did not want to miss a minute of his life.

Now I'm lying in this hospital dealing with what they tell me could be the end of my life, and he cannot be with me. Kids of his age are major germ carriers and, with my compromised immune system, they wouldn't let him be with me.

Only 10 minutes away, and he might as well be on the moon. I would look at the pictures of Christopher that I brought with me from my wallet at home. I would look at those pictures and my heart would just ache. Ache because he was not there and ache because I may not get the chance to raise him. And that's the deal I asked God to make with me, let me raise my son please.

Tick tock . . . only time will tell . . . tick tock

Chapter 19

In moments of discouragement, defeat, or even despair, there are always certain things to cling to.

Little things usually: remembered laughter, the face of a sleeping child, a tree in the wind - in fact, any reminder of something deeply felt or dearly loved.

No man is so poor as not to have many of these small candles.

When they are lighted, darkness goes away-and a touch of wonder remains."

~ *"These Small Candles" ...tombstone inscription in Britain*

Did Not Want Him to Worry

I wanted to live, not for me, but for Christopher. It was only a few months until his seventh birthday. Would I still be here to plan his party?

I had to figure out how to deal with the new reality of my life, at least what was to be left of it. I did not want Christopher to worry about me. That was much easier in the beginning, before the chemotherapy started to do a number on my body. It started with losing my hair, about two weeks after the first round of chemotherapy Christopher and I invited my nephew, "Little" Dan and his two kids to join us for a camping trip on the Oregon Coast.

Camping trips were something that Christopher and I loved doing. The first father-son trip that he and I took after I filed for divorce was a camping trip. We went to Jedediah Smith Redwoods State Park on the Smith River in northern California. But this trip was to the Oregon dunes. We stayed at Honeyman Memorial State Park.

My nephew is about six feet tall and well built. But his father was named Dan as well, so all my life I have known my nephew as "Little Dan" a name he no longer receives with the same smile he did when he *was* little. His kids, Aidan and Emmy Rose are just a little younger than Christopher and they always have a good time when they get together, which with such busy lives is just never often enough. This time though, we pulled it off, the five of us for a few days camping on the coast.

For those of you who have never had the pleasure of camping on the Oregon Coast you should know that you will be blessed with some truly beautiful days, but you can occasionally encounter some rain. It does not matter the season, rain can find you. I don't mind it, but just as air mattresses are not made for overnight sleeping, tents are not made for camping in the rain.

My body would no longer take sleeping on the ground in a tent like we used to do. No matter how much we spent on an inflatable mattress it always seemed to deflate during the night depositing me on a rock that was poking me in the most annoying way. So I broke down and bought a used trailer, 24 feet long and fully self-contained. No more late night dashes in the rain to the bathroom with a toddler in tow, screaming, "Dad I can't hold it any longer!"

This trip found Christopher and me getting to the campground early on Friday with a chance to set up camp before it got dark. Little Dan and his kids had to come over after he got off work, so they rolled in about nine that night. While Dan got his tent set up, Christopher showed the kids the lay of our camp. S'mores were made (they are mandatory, aren't they?) and consumed with enthusiasm and off to bed they all went.

Little Dan and I talked by the fire for a while and the subject of my hair came up. I was wearing a ball cap, but you could clearly see that I still had a head of hair. He asked, "How come your hair didn't fall out yet?" I told him, "I don't know," as I took off my cap. I grabbed a hand full of hair and I wondered out loud, "What, you think it should just come out?" To my surprise, it did!! I pulled my hand away from my head and out came a handful of hair. I looked at it for a few minutes and then tossed it into the fire, I grabbed another handful just to see, and sure enough it came out with no resistance. I thought about it for a minute, while Dan was explaining how gross that was, and I put my cap back on.

Losing my hair never really bothered me, I know it's a big deal for women; it's a part of how they see themselves. Luckily for me it was no big deal; other than the fact that my head was cold, I never gave it much thought.

This campground had a nice bathroom and shower set up - just keep pushing the button and hot water will continue as long as you wish. Good thing to know on a day where your bones might get cold on the Oregon Coast, but also a good thing when you are slowly removing your hair, handful after handful. Christopher and I spent more than our fair share of time in the shower together that next morning. Christopher was so intent on pushing that button he never said a word about my hair or the fact that it seemed to just wash away that morning.

I had explained to Christopher that, because of the chemotherapy, my hair would fall out. I shared with him that it was OK because when we were all done it would grow back. Some people said that it would even be better than before, darker, fuller and that area on top that somehow had thinned without my knowledge or consent would fill back in . . . Cool. I guess he got the message or perhaps my lack of hair was just no match for that button.

A thing about that shower button, Christopher never wanted to take a shower, but once he got in as long as he could push the button he would stay in forever. I had to fight to get him in and fight to get him out. It is the same to this day, go figure!

We all had a great time, we played on the dunes and we rode bikes around camp and went for walks. We drove over to the Sea Lion Caves, a great stop along the coast where thousands of loud barking sea lions hang out year round. From the gift shop at the top you work your way down the trail into the cave almost to sea level to get an up-close and personal look at (and smell of) way too many sea lions. Then you get to hike back up, oh joy!

Hiking down to the Sea Lion Caves was more painful and difficult than I thought it would be but the hike back up was near impossible to bear. I asked Little Dan to go ahead with the kids. I did not want to scare them or worry them, and it's so hard for me to have people watching while I just bawl like a baby, it hurts so, so bad.

As our camping trip drew to an end, Dan and his kids had to get back early so they headed out not long after breakfast on Sunday. Christopher and I headed over to the dunes, where we rented a dune buggy. It was a red two seater that would fly over the dunes if you let it. Yes, we flew more than a time or two. The problem was the dune buggy fit Christopher just fine, but I am 6'3" and with the mandatory helmet, my head hit the roll cage. I had to hold my head off center a little, which I did, but every time we hit a stiff bump or landed one of those fly-over's that Christopher loved so much, my head would hit . . . Ouch, but his laughter made it all worthwhile.

I think I still feel the pain of bouncing along the dunes especially the landings… no words to truly convey how much it hurt. So why do it? Because I can still see the smile on Christopher's face and his laughter of pure joy still rings in my ears.

When we were finally done with our aerial tricks, we headed back to camp. We had a meal, took yet another nap, then packed up the trailer and headed home. Smiles on our faces and new stories to share, there is no way to love more than I love my son. As I watched him sleep on the ride back home, I could not help but think about how much he meant to me and I wondered, I couldn't stop wondering if I would still be here for his next birthday.

The times that I could get out of bed to do these adventures, I did the best I could to hide the pain and fatigue. Forcing Christopher to take naps helped me a little because I usually got more sleep than he did. When it comes to driving, by the time I get to the 45-minute mark the pain is bad enough to make me cry, even with a full dose of narcotics. Most of those times even my best willpower couldn't hide the tears.

Why do these things… why put myself through it? There is no point being alive if I can't live… *truly* live life!

Chapter 20

The greatest loss of time is delay and expectation, which depend upon the future. We let go the present, which we have in our power, and look forward to that which depends upon chance, and so relinquish a certainty for an uncertainty.

~ Seneca

Round Two:
Remember, It's Going To Come Out!

I thought it was hard the first time I had to go into the hospital for chemo voluntarily. The first time, I had the fear of the unknown and all of the baggage from movies and stories we all hear. Not this time. This time I knew exactly what I was getting myself into. Why not add yet another issue, though? I am not sure what, but some part of the treatments had affected my blood sugar level, so in addition to all of the other drugs being put into my body, I was now on sliding-scale insulin injections. Just another prick or two in my day.

During my first round, I had survived what my oncologist's notes call severe nausea and emesis. So severe that he put together an aggressive treatment plan that would hopefully allow me at least some level of comfort. In addition to everything else, he added Anzemet with Decadron, Reglan (more about this one later), Benadryl, Compazine and Marinol.

Yes, that Marinol. THC, the active ingredient in pot, weed. All the benefits without lighting up and taking a puff on that magic dragon. Some people were excited to hear about this one. How did it make you feel, did you get high (No), did it give you the munchies? (No)

Are you kidding me? With all that was coming out, there was no interest in putting anything in. You actually learn to choose your food more wisely. Not from the normal standpoint of what sounds good, or what I would enjoy eating. No, your main consideration is "How will that feel coming out?" Major changes in eating habits right away!

So on May 31st at about seven in the morning, I presented myself for Round Two of chemotherapy. Fool me once, shame on you; fool me twice, shame on me. "Yes, Mr. Koop, you do have to check in at seven a.m. The delay last time was unusual, probably because it was your first time."

I know better now. Why? Because again, the chemotherapy did not start until about 6 to 7 p.m. that evening! To this day no one has explained it to me. I can hazard a few guesses, but I still don't really know why I got to spend all day waiting in a hospital bed again.

But treatment time finally rolled around. Same chemo drugs and those very same hazmat suits but this time I was ready, no surprise.

I've shared with you how hard it was for me that Christopher could not be with me during these chemotherapy treatments. I will tell you that with all this time to think I had another concern – a distant second, but a concern nonetheless. That's the fact that I was alone.

Here I was at what could be the end of my life and I was alone, no partner standing by my side. No one to hold me and tell me everything would be okay. No one I could count on to be there with me, no matter where my road went. All the people I had known, girlfriends and even a couple of wives, but here I was, all alone. At that moment I realized that I did not want my life to end this way. Somewhere out there was my soul mate, and if God gave me a chance I would work hard to find her.

Another new word, Zofran. "Zofran is my friend" is a little phrase I learned rather quickly! It is yet another anti-nausea drug. It comes in several forms, and the most effective for me was the one that instantly dissolved on my tongue. They only let me have it when I was out of the hospital. I looked forward to it as my "going away present." If I felt nausea coming on, Zofran would stop it, as long as I got it on my tongue before I actually started to vomit. If I was a moment too late, it offered no help at all.

I learned that the hospital waits until your nausea stops for 24 hours before they will release you to go home after chemo. A day free of gut wrenching spasms and upheaval and you are good to go. Whether you have the strength to go is not the question. It can't be. Fatigue and weakness are an ever-growing side effect of my chemotherapy treatments.

Neulasta is a shot that is given after each round of chemotherapy as needed. It is designed to increase your red cell blood count, in an effort to allow you to survive. The last time I heard, the cost is about $4,500 for each shot. But without it I would just become a lifeless puddle on the ground.

Five days after my admission for Round 2, on June 4th, I was released. Home again, with Tito, Rae (my other caregiver) and my Zofran by my side to take care of me.

I have known Rae and her family for about fifteen years. Rae worked with her family in their Christmas tree business. Because of Churchill and my other Christmas related businesses we would meet regularly at trade shows several times a year. Since their business and homes were in the same city as mine, we would see each other throughout the year.

Rae's dad Ernie had just gone through a battle with cancer and a drug trial. Rae was there to help with his care. So when I got sick she jumped right in and offered her help. She was just in-between houses so she moved into one of the guest bedrooms. Rae was a major part in my surviving Chemo. Thank You… Rae.

Chapter 21

Life is not about waiting for the storms to pass...
It's about learning how to dance in the rain.

~ Vivian Greene

The Toes Knows

During the course of my treatment I had gotten used to the idea of things feeling different or strange. Sometimes my body hurt and sometimes it was just different. On this day, it was strange and it was my toes. They didn't really hurt but I knew something was wrong. I took off my shoes, I was wearing those run faster, jump higher Nikes and my white socks at the toe were no longer white. They were soaked red with blood.

As you might guess, this caused me quite a bit of concern. So I called my doctor's office and explained the situation, asking if they could get me in straightaway. The staff at Dr. Kelber's office knew me well enough that if I called with a concern there was actually something wrong that needed to be dealt with, so they got me in pronto!

I learned a new phrase that day "spontaneous bleeding." Spontaneous bleeding falls into that category of new things I've learned that I wish I did not know. I will tell you that it's quite disconcerting to see blood leaking out of your toes without having smashed them or cut them, just because.

Dr. Kelber tells me there's not really a whole lot we can do at this point. We cannot dramatically change my dose of Coumadin. And there is very little to be done with the bleeding. The hope was that just as magically as the bleeding had spontaneously started, that it would quit. So I decided not to wear those shoes anymore and to limit my walking.

The next day found me wearing a really nice pair of "beach sandals." (Not a look I normally go for!) This change seemed to help reduce the bleeding in all except my big toe on my left foot. Anybody who was familiar with this syndrome and my doctor, who saw it, all believed that I would most likely lose the nail on my big toe, but it had not yet come off. The problem was it had become infected.

Dr. Kelber gave me antibiotics in order to try to clear up the infection. The first round did not seem to work and so the decision was to do a stronger course of antibiotics and, if that did not work, to go with direct injections. At this point he explained to me that if they could not get the infection under control they would have to amputate. Here we go once again, big choices. Big toe or no big toe? Left foot or no left foot? It just seemed like sometimes it never ends.

When I got home I fell down on the bed and I cried. I asked the question that I asked a few times before that and many times since "When is enough, enough?"

I am happy to say that the second course of antibiotics took care of the infection and the big toe on my left foot is still in place. It did take another 18 months for the toenail to come all the way off and it still has yet to grow all the way back.

Chapter 22

It is good to have an end to journey toward, but it is the journey that matters in the end.

~ Ursula K. LeGuin

Round Three:
Goodbye to the Gold Wing

So here we are. It's June 21, 2006, and for the third time I'm be-ing asked to voluntarily make my way to the hospital for round three of my chemotherapy. Each round is proving to be more difficult than the previous one. My energy level is down, and the pain and fatigue is increasing every week.

This is the end of the first half of the treatment plan developed by Dr. Ryan at OHSU and Dr. Pierce at Salem Hospital. It called for three rounds of chemotherapy. Then after enough time went by for me to rebuild my strength, I'd have surgery to remove the base of my spine. Once I recovered from surgery sufficiently to withstand it – that's right, three more rounds of chemotherapy to follow up.

Once again, I suffered from severe and prolonged, intractable nausea and vomiting during round two of chemotherapy. My weak-ness and fatigue was a growing concern. I began to lose weight at an alarming rate. I have always been a big man, and prior to getting cancer my top weight was 302 pounds. Standing 6' 3" I carried it well, but it had steadily been going down since I had gotten sick. I was now down to 250 pounds, a loss of 52 pounds.

My hospital room was still empty. Luckily, the meds they were giving me put me to sleep much of the time. But when I was awake I was still haunted by the same concerns: missing Christopher and the thought of dying alone. And now I was unable to put the upcoming surgery out of my mind. The results are designed to let me survive this cancer, but the cost to my day-to-day life is going to be cata-strophic. The results of the surgery might include a colostomy bag and the need for a wheelchair, as the doctors expected I would be paralyzed from the waist down.

Christopher was not sure what to think about this, not sure that it was anything good. I took the time to try to turn it around, to make it fun in his mind, something to actually look forward to. "What are we going to do, Dad?" he asked.

I said, "Well, first we get to go out and buy a new car! One of those cool vans, the ones that come with a ramp. The ones that have pedals for the gas and brakes on the steering wheel. That way I can still drive. Then we get to pick out a four wheel drive wheelchair." He thought that was exciting and wanted to know if he could drive the wheelchair, too. "Absolutely," I told him.

There was one thing though, knowing myself as well as I do, that I don't think I could have dealt with. That was my Honda Gold Wing Aspencade. I have ridden motorcycles most of my adult life and this was my fourth Gold Wing. If I was to come home from the hospital in that wheelchair and had to come face to face with my bike just sitting there in my garage, knowing that I could no longer ride, it would have been too much for me.

So I sold my Gold Wing, making sure that I had nothing to freak out about when I got home. It was a sad day for me but it was something that I had to do. Once I came to grips with the fact that I would have to sell my Gold Wing, I placed an ad on Craig's list. I started to get calls fairly quickly and one man and his wife came out the very next day. They seemed nice enough and liked the bike. He asked if he could take it for a test drive and I told him "No." I explained that it's my bike until someone buys it, and I never let anyone ride my bike. You never know what might happen.

He was insulted that I was questioning his ability to ride. I explained that it was not personal, I was sure that he had the experience that he said he did, but no one rides my bike, period. If you like my bike and you want to buy it, put the money, cash not check, on the table and you can go for a ride on your new bike. If for any reason the bike is not exactly like I said, and if you find a problem, I'll give you your money back. I explained it would all be in writing on the bill of sale – that way we are both covered.

He did not like it but he agreed to gather the money and come back the next day. He did indeed show up the next day, along with three cars full of assorted people who accompanied him. Turns out he was the minister of a small church and his birthday was coming up. The parishioners of his church, along with his wife and kids, had raised a collection to buy him the bike for his birthday. They all looked over the bike and agreed that they should buy it.

Each person produced various envelopes of cash, and shortly thereafter I had my money and they had a beautiful Gold Wing. I started to go around the bike in an effort to show him all the features of the bike. He became very indignant and repeated that he had 25 years of experience and he "did not need me to show him anything, OK?" He was flat out rude to me and repeated that he didn't need anyone to tell him about riding a bike. At the risk of being chastised again, I made one more suggestion. A trailer was included in the deal so I suggested that I could disconnect it, and he could go for a short ride to get used to the bike before he headed out with the trailer in tow (he had shared with me that he had never pulled a trailer behind a bike).

He agreed and we unhooked the trailer and everyone in his entourage left, except his wife. He headed out the driveway and down the hill to the highway. About ten minutes later his wife's cell phone rang. She answered it, listened for a while and then said, "I don't understand." She repeated it several times, "I don't understand, I don't understand." Finally I interrupted and asked if everything was OK? She said to me that he is trying to explain that he totaled the bike. What?? Trying to get my brain around what was happening, I asked, "Is he OK?" She looked at me and repeated into the phone again... "I don't understand what you are telling me." I repeated my question, "Is he OK? Do we need to call 911?"

Her husband was calling to say that he had been in an accident, that he totaled the bike. She appeared to be so concerned about the bike that she and the parishioners had just bought, that she could not bother to ask if HE was OK! Finally she said to me that he was partway down the hill, he had never even made it to the highway. This man with over 25 years of experience drove his Gold Wing (not mine) over the bank of the road. I jumped into my truck and asked her to get in; she said no I am going to wait here. I drove down the hill and found him standing on the side of the road looking over the edge at his brand new Gold Wing. He had some scrapes and bruises but I believe the greatest damage was to his ego. How does that saying go? Pride Goethe Before a Fall? Once I was sure that he was indeed OK, that saying just kept repeating in my head.

That is exactly why no one ever rides my bike . . . you just never know!

When the paralysis and wheelchair topic came up at OHSU, I was told that I needed to get counseling. "No," I said, "I don't think so." The doctors explained that this would be a major life-changing event, something that I should get in front of, and learn how to deal with the upcoming changes. Serious depression is a normal response to finding yourself stuck in a wheel chair. Sometimes you begin to think that life is not worth living. It was easy for me, if my choices were to be dead from this cancer and not get to raise my son or get to raise him, but from a chair. It was a no-brainer for me. No, I did not want to be in a wheelchair for the rest of my life, but if that's what it took to get to raise my son, then so be it.

Round Three was a doozy and it was 10 days before I was discharged from Salem Hospital. I was weak as a human could be and still be alive. Discharged and sent home to gain strength so that I could undergo the surgery that would change my life forever. Survive the surgery or not, colostomy bag or not, paralysis or not.

Tick tock, only time would tell (and that's what I had, time with nothing to do but think about it), tick tock, tick tock.

Chapter 23

Traveling is not just seeing the new; it is also leaving behind. Not just opening doors; also closing them behind you, never to return. But the place you have left forever is always there for you to see whenever you shut your eyes.

~ Jan Myrdal

Shamu . . . Up Close and Personal!

Dr. Krajbich's assistant, Amy, was the person I spent most of my time with at OHSU. She was very good at her job, comforting, and knowledgeable in all aspects of my treatment.

All of my chemotherapy treatments were performed at Salem Hospital, so I could be close to my home and family. That also allowed me to continue my daily care with my oncologist, Dr. Pierce since his office is in Salem Hospital's Center for Outpatient Medicine, the COM building on their campus. He just had a short walk over the sky bridge and a couple of elevator rides to do rounds on 5 south, the cancer wing.

So there I was, at OHSU after round three of chemotherapy for a status update with Amy and Dr. Krajbich. A new MRI was done so that we had current film on the status of my cancer after three rounds of chemotherapy and the previous surgical biopsies. After a complete review, a short date was set for the resection. I hesitated and then asked how much, if any, damage would be done if we waited. They asked why I wanted to postpone the surgery. I explained that I wanted to take my son on a vacation.

It had been quite awhile since Christopher and I had had a chance to have some major fun, one-on-one father son time. I also was thinking about that damn wheel chair. I wanted to take one last vacation where I could walk, hold my son's hand and walk side by side as we laughed our way through yet another adventure. After this surgery, as long as I survived it, life by itself, let alone traveling, was going to be more difficult. I just wanted one more trip . . . to build one more memory with my son.

The doctors gave me the OK as long as I could schedule the trip right away . . . Orbitz.com, here I come! I made reservations for a trip to San Diego's Sea World. We were both very excited and looked forward to the trip. Secretly I was concerned about traveling, and trying to keep up with a seven year old. My pain level was high, my energy level was low, and it did not take much to induce vomiting.

Each step of the way good things happened to us that made things easier or just more fun. At the airport the nice lady who handled our check-in at the Alaska Airlines counter could tell just by looking at me that I was in a bad way, she asked if I was OK. I explained about the cancer and the surgery that awaited our return, about my desire to build positive loving memories for my son . . . I could see the tears forming in her eyes. When she handed me our new boarding passes I saw that she had upgraded us to first class, so kind and thoughtful.

Apparently she had put a note in the record for the crew on the plane because they fawned over Christopher. He got to hang out with the pilot in the cockpit during boarding. He is a super smart kid and always wants to know how things work, lots of great questions and paying oh so close attention to the answers. They also did their best to make me comfortable. Alaska Airlines . . . Thank you from the bottom of my heart.

When we landed in San Diego and stopped at the car rental area, Christopher caught sight of a bright yellow Hummer H3 by the door to the counter. Once again it was impossible for the man at the counter not to notice that I was seriously ill. Once again I explained about my cancer, the surgery that awaited us upon my return, and my effort to build memories with my son. Several times during our conversation, Christopher shared his desire to travel the road ahead of us in that bright yellow Hummer H3. I have to admit it looked very cool, but our reservation was for a $15.00 a day small car. The man at the counter explained several times, almost like he felt guilty about it that our reservation would not allow for an upgrade without paying many hundreds of dollars extra.

I asked Christopher, "Do you want to spend all that money for the upgrade, or would you like to save it for souvenirs and other things that we might find that we would want to take home with us?" He made the hard choice to pass on the Hummer. The young man at the counter then excused himself for a minute. He came back with a man who he introduced as his manager. The manager took his measure of Christopher and me, and then he asked Christopher if he really, really wanted to hit the highway in that way cool, bright yellow Hummer? Yes, absolutely yes was his reply. It happened once again, they gave us the upgrade (at no cost) to help me build those memories. So with smiles on our faces and thanks in our hearts we made our way to our hotel, in our bright yellow Hummer H3.

The next day we got up and made our way to Sea World. Mornings are usually hard for me, so by the time we got there it was late morning and all of the wheelchairs were gone. I was not sure that I could keep up with Christopher, so I had called ahead during the planning stages and found out that they provided wheelchairs. During the discussions with Sea World that morning about the chairs, or lack thereof, they learned about what I was trying to do, and they decided to help. They provided us with a personal escort for the day, expediting our way through lines to help me. Giving us some looks behind the scenes, it was very special treatment that helped to create the kind of special memories I was looking for. It was the final thing that Maggie, our private tour guide arranged that put our experience over the top. The last show that we went to was "Believe," the Shamu show.

Maggie had arranged for Christopher to be called up from the audience to be part of the team of trainers. He got to meet Shamu up close and personal. He got to go down to the deck at the edge of the pool to pet and feed Shamu a snack of stinky fish. As he lined up with the other trainers his picture was shown large on the JumboTron. The trainers gave him a souvenir necklace with a whale's tail to memorialize his time with Shamu . . . Talk about memories, thank you Maggie, thank you trainers and thank you Sea World!

As with all of our other adventures and day-to-day life, I worked hard on this trip to hide the pain so that Christopher and anyone else near us would not have to worry about me.

Chapter 24

Today is the tomorrow we worried about yesterday.

~ Author Unknown

The Watermelon Slice

Three times in a row I took the trip from home to Salem Hospital. A 15-minute ride to voluntarily face chemotherapy. Those rides seemed to last forever, until this day. I was riding in the passenger seat, headed north on I-5. My head was resting against the door window as I tried not to think about what was to come. Somehow that only seemed to focus my mind on what I was trying to avoid . . . My life was only a few hours from changing completely as I knew it.

It's only an hour drive to OHSU, but I was traveling a lifetime. Every time you go in for major surgery the consent forms always include the possibility of death, but that's not what worried me. This time the results are likely: paralysis, joined by a colostomy bag, impotence and incontinence of the bowels and the bladder. My mind bounced back and forth from all the active things I'd done in the past, and all the things that I wouldn't be able to do in the future. This ride will take away my freedom, my ability to walk and run, my ability to be a man. This was the longest hour I had ever spent. I didn't really want it to end. When this ride was over, life as I knew it would be over too.

Just like showing up for chemo at the Salem Hospital, when I finally get to OHSU and settled in my room, I had to wait and wait and then wait some more. Rae was my chauffeur for the ride up and she was sitting quietly by my side. I have never met any other human being who can be happy, completely happy just sitting quietly for hours on end. In this case, that was mostly a good thing. There was nothing I could think of that I wanted to talk about. Right then, I wished I could just turn my brain off.

A hypodermic needle full of something good had just been injected into my IV and my mind began to drift off. I think I remember telling Rae goodbye, but I'm not sure. The next thing I remember is waking up, that's right, I'm awake so I guess I did not die on the table.

While I was on the table Dr. Krajbich and his team worked their magic. Every time a biopsy was done, there was a chance that cancer cells could be spread to a different part of my body. With every open surgical biopsy that was done, the chance of spreading those cancer cells increased. So with this resection of my sacrum, they took out a wedge-shaped portion of my backside, outside the margins of all previous surgeries and biopsies in an effort to ensure that all cancer cells were removed. I thought of it like a great big wedge of watermelon at the Fourth of July Barbecue. Now I can truly use those "Half Assed" jokes.

It only takes one little guy to jump on the bloodstream highway, stopping wherever he chooses to establish what they call a metastasis, where the cancer spreads to other parts of your body. Each and every time they did a biopsy, or an open surgical biopsy, it was like stirring up a hornet's nest of cancer cells – where did they all go? With a normal biopsy the doctor would use a small needle or a punch to take a very small sample, from not very deep, to all the way to the bone. With an open surgical biopsy, I was placed under general anesthesia and opened up, way up with a scalpel. Large amounts of tissue and bone samples were removed. Having a wide open field of view gives the surgeon a good look at what is really going on in there, and what he wants to remove portions of to get the best biopsy results. Great for the biopsy, but a greater risk each time for the possibility of spreading the cancer cells.

Once Dr. Krajbich and his team had worked their way down through tissue and muscle, all the while dealing with a tangle of nerves coming out of my spine, they were able to use a bone saw to cut off my sacrum, that triangle bone between your pelvic bones. I don't have one of those anymore. All of the tissue to a margin just outside of all previous biopsies and surgeries was removed. Then they had to put me back together again, working their way back up to the surface. They used a cool type of netting, called Mersilene mesh, to provide the support internally where the bone used to be. That netting now holds it all in place.

Date: Thu, 27 Jul 2006 11:55:19 -0700
From: Jody
Subject: Re: David update
To: Janene

David had his surgery on Friday, July 21, 2006. After 3 rounds of chemo it was surgery time. They removed the lower part of his spine. Because of where it was and what was connected we were really worried. But I talked to him Sunday and he said I can See, I am not blind, I have no colon bag and I can wiggle my toes. He was so happy. He was still on morphine, but it is good. Prayer works. There is still 3 more rounds of chemo to go and I say thumbs up!!

I will update as we go.

Love Jody

Date: Sun, 30 Jul 2006 09:08:32 -0700
From: DAK
To: "DAK (E-mail)"

Subject:

YA HOOOOOOOOOOOOOOOOOOOOOOOOOOOOOOOOOOO !!!!! !!!!! !!!!

I was released from OHSU on Friday... one week after the operation.

Same joy as last time... I could see!!! I could move my toes!!! No bag hanging off my side!!!!

I think I now know why I don't win the lotto... God has been saving up my luck for this!

By the power of all your prayers and a great surgeon I am doing amazingly well !

There are some nerve issues we are waiting to see about along with a couple of other things but all in all I am one of the luckiest and happiest people you will ever know.

Love you all... David

As happy as I was about the great results, the recovery was more difficult this time, much harder and more painful than before. The pain meds finally got dialed in to where I was at least a little comfortable. When out of the blue, and for no good reason, one of the doctors who came in the middle of the night changed my pain meds. He changed them from meds that were working to an entirely different medication that just did not touch my pain. I woke up crying out in pain.

I was so fearful. I had no idea that my meds had been changed. All I knew was that the pain was getting worse and worse. It had become unbearable! What was happening to me? Finally, one of the nurses discovered that my pain meds had been changed in the middle of the night. Once the problem was found it seemed to take forever to get my meds changed back. When they finally got the old meds back on orders it seemed to take a lifetime to get the excruciating pain under control. I have no idea why that doctor decided to change my meds without talking to me. But it was the worst decision involved in my care.

Just seven days after my ride north to OHSU, and I was headed home after making my way to the car under my own power. Who would've thought walking? I still can't believe how lucky I am. The ride home is full of my future, I am still alive, and I am walking. I am planning in my head for the future... my future.

Thank you, OHSU. Thank you Dr. Krajbich and all of your team. Without your skills and dedication my life would be so different.

What does my future hold? Only time will tell.

Tick tock . . . only time will tell . . . tick tock

Chapter 25

A smile costs nothing, but gives much. It enriches those who receive, without making poorer those who give. It takes but a moment, but the memory of it sometimes lasts forever. None is so rich or might that he can get along without it and none is so poor that he can be made rich by it. A smile creates happiness in the home, fosters good will in business, and is the countersign of friendship. It brings rest to the weary, cheer to the discouraged, sunshine to the sad, and it is nature's best antidote for trouble. Yet it cannot be bought, begged, borrowed, or stolen, for it is something that is of no value to anyone until it is given away. Some people are too tired to give you a smile. Give them one of yours, as none needs a smile so much as he who has no more to give.

~ Author Unknown

Round Four:
Can I Really Take Any More?

August 24, 2006: my doctors concluded that I had healed enough from my surgery that the fourth round of chemotherapy could be started.

So there I was, preparing to start round four of chemotherapy. This time it was different, very different from my previous chemotherapy treatments. Gone was my energy level; gone was the joking, jovial patient. The previous rounds of chemotherapy and the tremendous stress on my body and my mind from my most recent surgery had left me just a shell of my former self.

It was almost like an out-of-body experience. I knew that my body was going through this but I seemed to be off hovering in a corner somewhere. I knew what was happening, it just wasn't happening to me. It was surreal.

The emesis and the complete lack of hunger had me down to 230 pounds, 72 pounds from my high. Eating was just something that I did not want to do. A simple drink of water could start the vomiting . . . *Zofran, where is my Zofr . . . Too late . . .*

Milkshakes and fruit smoothies with yogurt are some of the things we tried. Because of Christopher's potentially fatal peanut allergy, no peanut products have been allowed in the house for years. But they are a good source of protein, and the doctors wanted me to try eating them. Rae put together a clean zone in the laundry room, plastic down on the counter, paper plates, plastic knives. It all got thrown away. Nothing could remain in the house or go in the dishwasher because the peanut antigen could transfer. Nothing peanut related can ever get to Christopher.

What I found, by accident, was that food from the restaurant *Mount Fuji Rice Time* worked for me. As soon as it seemed that I might be able to eat, I tried a bowl of miso soup and was able to keep it down. As I got stronger, I added a California roll and finally a few days later I was able to add a shrimp tempura roll. I told the owners that their food was my "cancer medicine."

The owners were very sweet. It was obvious by looking at me that I was sick. First they noticed that I could not hold the chop sticks like I used to. The woman owner came over and whispered in my ear, "Use your fingers, it is okay, you need food, just pick it up." Then I would be gone for weeks at a time before showing up again.

"Where have you been?" she asked. I told her that I had been back in the hospital for more chemotherapy. She said, "Oh, their food is no good, next time you call and I bring you food."

She did not really know me. I had not eaten there that often in the past, but she just genuinely cared about another human being. I only took her up on the free food and delivery to the hospital once. But her food was the magic medicine that helped me to regain my strength each time I completed a round of chemotherapy. Many times my caregivers and friends would just laugh because, when they went to pick up takeout for me, all they had to do was say "they needed the food for that big cancer guy," and everyone at the restaurant knew who I was. Not only did they know the order, but they always made it special, with extra shrimp and avocado on the outside of my California roll, and they never billed me the full amount, if at all.

There are truly nice people in this world of ours, offering random acts of kindness. That's something I have always tried to practice, but I had no idea how good it felt to be on the receiving end!

I had to get my strength back, the good food was helping, but I was so very tired and so very sick. When would I turn the corner?

Tick tock . . . only time will tell . . . tick tock

Chapter 26

The only thing that makes life possible is permanent, intolerable uncertainty; not knowing what comes next.

~ Ursula K. LeGuin

Mirror Mirror on the Wall . . . OMG!

A few days after being released from my fourth round of chemotherapy, I took a short walk. The same walk I had taken hundreds of times before, but this time I caught something in my peripheral vision. It stopped me in my tracks. I moved back a step or two to get a better view. OMG . . . I can see some old man that looks like death warmed over. It instantly takes my mind back to the photos of men from the concentration camps. With pale whitish gray skin that seems to be falling off in patches and bones protruding in areas where bones have never been seen before. No hair anywhere in sight not even eyebrows, just a sunken pale gray orb where a head used to be.

He was not like death warmed over. As I looked at that man more closely, a truer vision came to be, he looked like death. As my mind came back to reality I realized that I was vomiting in the sink of my master bathroom. I looked up and saw the wall-to-wall mirror before me and then I knew: it was me. I had just caught the first true glimpse of what had happened to my body and to me. I had been surviving the truth by hiding from it, but here I was face-to-face with my new reality. I cried at what I saw. It actually made me sick, like I needed another reason to get sick?

One of my caregivers covered that mirror so that I would not have to spend time with that man. He was someone else's reality, in my mind I survived knowing who I was, a strong mountain of a man. As time went on and I became stronger in mind and body, that mirror was uncovered and the sight of that man, as I passed by, no longer made me want to puke.

They say you have to hit bottom to get better, I guess that was my bottom. I actually had no idea who that man in the mirror was when he first came into view. Upon focusing I realized it was my body, but it was not me. It was not who I had been as a man and it was not who I would be. I would do whatever was in my power to get better, to get me back to the man I know I am.

Chapter 27

If you're going through hell, keep going.

~ Winston Churchill

Round Five:
If Only I Can Survive!

September 20th, 2006: Not really sure how I got here. Who brought me to Five South yet again? My body knows the drill, but my mind just cannot focus. I can't do this anymore and yet I still have at least two more rounds to go.

Things were not going well. In fact, things were going downhill quickly. This was not the same as my previous rounds.

I had a port that was surgically installed in my upper left chest when we started chemo so that they would not have to establish an IV site each time. Unfortunately, there was a new drug that had to be put into my body but it could not come in contact with the chemotherapy drugs in my existing mainline port. Yes, I know, I asked the same question . . . The chemotherapy drugs are going into my blood stream and all over my body, right? This new drug is going into my blood stream and all over my body as well, right? They explained it's just a timing thing. In the body okay, in the IV tube not good at all.

It was late afternoon or early evening and they needed to establish a new IV. The nurse came in and she was unable to hit the vein, so she tried again. Her second attempt failed, so she moved to a new site. Strike three! She wanted to try again at yet another site, but I politely said, "Three strikes and you are out." It hurt more than normal and I had lost confidence in her.

I asked her if we really needed to have this drug now. Can't we just wait? "No," she said, "you need it now." I politely asked her to get someone else to establish my IV. A little later, another nurse came in, and along with the first nurse they apologized for putting me through this but they would get it done.

After demonstrating *her* inability to establish an IV the second nurse finally said, well I am going to call IV services. They specialized in difficult cases, since we were on to our fifth attempt (yes the fourth missed the mark as well), we needed their special skills. Because of the previous missed attempts the best spot available was now on my hand, on the back near the edge. I had one there once before and did not like it. The previous time it hurt going in, it was painful the entire time while it was there, and it always seemed to be catching on things, jamming it this way and that. No fun at all.

The specialist from IV services said if this site failed she had another site that she could try. I explained in no uncertain terms that it would not be an issue. I would not allow a sixth attempt. I didn't care how bad I need it. I was done for the night. Get it on this try or wait until tomorrow. God decided I had endured enough over a simple IV. The fifth time was a charm. It may not seem like much but there I was on my fifth round of chemo, sick and tired, everything hurt. To top it off I had become a human pin cushion. It was just too much that day. What could be next? I'd had enough already.

My insides were coming out. The chemo drugs were literally burning up my insides. I was coughing up blood, and tissue was coming out the other end as the treatment was literally burning off my insides. A painful disgusting chemical burn and I agreed to it. I gave them permission to do this to me.

Then there were the results of my current blood work. Not good, not good at all. My creatinine numbers were down, way down! So what did it mean? It meant that if my numbers didn't come back up . . . dialysis on a regular basis until a new kidney could be found. That's right, a kidney transplant if a match could be found. How long do people wait for a match? How many people die each day waiting for a match that is never found? How many things can I deal with or think about, even worry about before my head just explodes?

Lasix, that's the newest member of my drug team. I was now suffering from fluid overload. Sounds so polite . . . *"fluid overload."* No worries though, the Lasix would take care of it. Fluid overload is when your body begins to retain fluids, so much so that you begin to swell up. If they are unable to get your body to expel those fluids your heart can stop and you can eventually drown in your own fluids. Come on Lasix!

What was happening? Something new . . . again. I woke up and I couldn't help but notice that my hands were shaking like a Parkinson's patient, uncontrollable shaking. What was happening? It seems that everything has been listed as a possible side effect of one drug or another, but no one ever said anything about this. Is it affecting my voice too? Or is it just my ears? Oh my God, am I going to be like this forever? Never holding a glass of water again, not able to write. Is it going to get worse?

Reglan is one of the many drugs I was getting. These were the possible side effects. Stop the drug and the symptoms should improve, that's what the doctors are telling me. Should?

Hell, it's not the cancer that will kill me – it's the treatment. People wonder (I know I did), can I survive this cancer? I am not really worrying about the cancer right now. I want to know if I can survive the treatment!

The treatment, right, the treatment. I need these drugs. The treatment plan required to help me beat this cancer. Six rounds of Adriamycin and Cisplatin, the oldest, meanest chemotherapy drugs a body can encounter.

OK, I give! And the doctors did too. They advised me that we will stop early, not even completing all of round five. The damage to my heart, damage to my kidneys, and God knows what else burned up inside me by these chemicals had been too great. My body couldn't take any more. Could I now believe that not even five complete rounds will do what I was told required six rounds to accomplish? First I had to hope and pray that I could survive six rounds of these chemotherapy drugs. Now I had to hope and pray that I could survive without six? Dr. Pierce was very clear, after looking at me and my labs that I was done with chemo.

Seven days after my body showed up at Five South, I am sent home again. Home was never a walk in the park. Each time I was released it was just as I barely had the strength to go. Many times the nausea was so bad that just the smell of water would start the vomiting.

I didn't know what was happening in the outside world. The world was continuing on without me. Would I ever rejoin the masses?

Tick tock . . . only time will tell . . . tick tock

Chapter 28

Whether seventy or sixteen, there is in every being's heart a love of wonder; the sweet amazement at the stars and starlike things and thoughts; the undaunted challenge of events, the unfailing childlike appetite for what comes next, and the joy in the game of life

~ Samuel Ullman

The Love of a Child

For different reasons and at different times, all parents struggle with, "Is my child ready to handle this information?" That question certainly came up for me, when the doctors and the tests told me that I would be dead before the end of the year.

There was no hiding from Christopher the fact that his Dad was sick. I was in and out of the doctor's office and in and out of the hospital time after time. My appearance was obviously changing. I had been telling the doctors and myself that despite their expertise, I was not conceding that I was going to die; as a matter of fact I was quite positive that I was not. But what do I tell my son?

When there were major changes I sat Christopher down, and we talked about the fact that I was sick and that I had cancer. I asked Christopher if he understood what cancer was. Not surprisingly at all, his understanding was quite accurate. But I did not tell him what the doctors were telling me – that I was likely going to die before his next birthday.

One day Christopher came into the master bedroom. I was in my usual place, flat on my back in the bed. He crawled up next to me, was talking about this and that, and he stopped and sat up on the bed. He looked at me and the next thing he said brought tears to my eyes.

My seven-year-old son said, "Dad, I don't want you to worry. I'm going to get married as fast as I can, and I'm going to have kids as quick as I can . . . so that you can have grandchildren."

He did not say the words, but they were hanging thick in the air . . . I want you to be with your grandkids. I want to give you grandkids, before you die. Through my tears I told him how much I loved him and how much that meant to me. I also explained to Christopher that he needed to take his time because I was planning on being around for a long time. And he needed to take the time to find the right woman that he could spend the rest of his life with and grandkids would follow naturally.

To this day my heart is warmed by the love of my son. How a seven-year-old got it into his head how valuable the gift of grand-children could be, I will never know. But it's not the first time he surprised me. It wasn't the last time, and I know even from this day forward, there will be many more times that my son surprises me with his insights on life.

Chapter 29

Being defeated is often a temporary condition. Giving up is what makes it permanent."

~ Marilyn Vos Savant

Round Six

Five times in a row I made the trip to present myself for the torture of chemotherapy. For number six I have been let off the hook. Instead of worrying what would happen to my body during round six, I instead find myself worrying about what will happen without it.

Did just one of those microscopic cancer cells get dislodged during all of those biopsies and surgeries? Has it set up a new home base, maybe in my lungs? Only time will tell for me. It's time to heal this battered body of mine, will I make it?

Tick tock . . . only time will tell . . . tick tock

Who knew that just about a year later, I'd be sending an email like this to my group:

Date: 26 Jul 2007
From: DAK
To: "DAK (E-mail)"
Subject:
ok… Ok… OK !

I hear you all; I have been very lack in disseminating information recently.

First I am not dead… Far from it (this is a good thing). I am getting stronger each week. It is very slow progress… but it is progress. When I look at where I was Last July, surgery that was to leave me paralyzed for life, to where I am now. I am without a doubt the luckiest man you know!!!

Christopher and I have been camping over at the coast; and we took a trip to Bend in our new Porsche Boxster. At the end of July we are going on a cruise! We are planning a driving trip to Yellowstone National Park at the end of august (after this last trip I am not completely sure about driving all that way), but we do look forward to seeing Bon and Ev again. I got to be the coach for Christopher's soccer team this spring... yea! I am also the newly elected Vice Chair of the Parent club at his school. I truly enjoyed the time I got to spend during 2007 as a parent teacher, working with Christopher and other kids in his class.

I still have some bad days... sometimes really, really bad days. But I get through them and they do not come as often. I have gained 27 of the 92 pounds that I lost and most of my hair is back. We put in a home gym to help rebuild all of the muscle that I lost. Christopher is a huge help; he loves doing it with me and eggs me on.

A few days ago I participated as one of the survivors at the American Cancer Society's "Relay for Life". It was a very moving, highly emotional day and evening. I hope to attend each year for a long time. And if I am gone I would love to know that someone is taking Christopher as part of a team raising money and doing laps in memory of me. I intend to add something about that to my will.

I love you all and I want to tell you again how much your thoughts, your prayers all the cards (even the goofy ones)... how much they all mean to me and how they have helped and do help in getting me through the dips in my road as I make this journey.

Thank you all... David

(Never got to make that trip to Yellowstone National Park, who was I kidding? Driving all the way to Yellowstone was just never in the cards.)

Chapter 30

I am determined to be cheerful and happy in whatever situation I may find myself. For I have learned that the greater part of our misery or unhappiness is determined not by our circumstance but by our disposition.

~ Martha Washington

Depression

Three years, four months and eleven days. That's how long it took from the morning when Dr. Kelber said, "It's bad, it is really bad news" until I felt like there was no point in going on any longer. I was thinking that being dead would be better than living.

Yes, there were times, during chemo, waiting for them to finally get a correct diagnosis, mostly when I looked at my son. Times, yes, there were times that I felt bad. It was depressing, but not capital "D" Depression.

The doctors all continued to offer antidepressants. They said it was normal, normal to be depressed, normal to need help getting through it. Help to try to stay sane, while you have no idea what's actually wrong, whether you will live or die, whether I would get to see my son grow up, whether I would get the chance to raise him. Whether I would get the chance to teach my son the things I knew, protect him from the bad things I knew about in the world. No way for there to be happy thoughts. Hell, it was all very depressing, but it was not Depression.

So what was different now? I'm not really sure. The only thing I can come up with is for three years, four months and eleven days, all that time, I hadn't been able to be ME.

I am unable to work. I have tried a couple of times. Starting off easy, or so I thought. Three hours per day, four days a week. I was helping Peak Seasons; they needed someone to run a warehouse distribution center in the Pacific Northwest.

My body simply would not allow me to do it. The pain was so severe that some days I could not get out of bed, pain so bad that it makes you vomit. Other days I was just physically unable to stay for the three hours I had committed to.

I have faced physical problems several times in my life, and I have always been able to deal with them and continue to improve my condition. My thoughts always stayed on message: I might be hurt and somewhat disabled now, but I'm going to do what it takes to get better!

I have never liked taking pain meds and have always worked hard to get off of them, even with this cancer. I was using the Fentanyl patch (100 times stronger than morphine), Neurontin, morphine and finally Oxycodone for breakthrough pain right after the surgery.

Even with all of these pain medications, I still had to deal with horrific pain regularly, causing me to spend most of my time in bed. I wanted to be up and active, but the more I did, the more I hurt. Even during the worst of it, though, what I was planning on was getting better.

I tried reducing the amount of medication I needed each day, always working towards the day when I could get back to the hardworking guy I used to be. Working hard to ensure that the special people in my life are happy and that they know how I feel about them, knowing that I will move mountains to ensure that they feel loved. Working hard at my whole life: The things I did to earn a living, working hard at the fun things I have enjoyed, travel, sailing, scuba diving, and so much more. Hell, I can't even take a long drive in the car any more.

The Fentanyl was first. My Fentanyl was a transdermal patch. I placed it high on the top of my shoulder. More than once I had a problem with the patch getting washed off or steamed off when I used the hot tub. The hot tub was so therapeutic I needed to continue using it each and every day. So I used positive mental imaging and biofeedback to get my brain and my body ready to dump the Fentanyl patch. It took a massive amount of willpower but I did it.

One down, three more to go, the Neurontin was next. I gradually reduced the amount I took, until one day I was able to stop taking it altogether. *Success!* I told myself. *Moving in the right direction. I am moving through this process, and I'm going to come out the other side, big, strong and ready to take on the world.*

Now, it was time for the morphine. Several times I tried to reduce the amount of morphine that I took each day, but I could not do it. Even worse for me was the new reality in my life. The more I did, the more I hurt.

When I say hurt, I don't mean, "You know, my back is kinda sore." No, I mean curled up in bed for two or three days. Curled up like a baby in the fetal position, screaming in pain and bawling like a child, knowing that it is so bad that I might not make it.

So I take the drugs, and lie in bed like a vegetable. When I get the strength, I get into the hot tub. Then I am ready to try again.

Unless you have been there, there is no way to know how much energy it takes just for me to act normal. To go to the Cub Scout meeting with Christopher, to help at his school, or to go have a meal with a friend.

Instead of reducing the morphine, the dose has actually increased and increased over time, all in an effort to achieve some quality of life. Forget about working, I'm just trying to live. Then the itching started . . . itching, itching!!!!

When I say itch, it is impossible for you to understand. I don't mean like I have a mosquito bite or a slight rash. I'm talking about that kind of itch that would drive most people completely insane. And I'm not exaggerating. I mean, if you don't have the strongest of mental capabilities, you would go crazy with this itch, and I got real close.

This is the kind of itch that gets so bad that you want to take a food grater or a knife and just cut it off, just get it away from your body, you just cannot stand it.

And that's what I did, I took a device, I think they call it a cuticle tool. This is an ergonomically designed plastic molded handle with a very sharp V shaped blade on the end of it. I took that tool and I carved my legs until the pain was greater than the itch. It's not something I'm proud of but I just couldn't stand it any longer. It was driving me crazy.

And we're adding this to the pain, the incontinence, the impotence and the ever-growing depression. This itch, it's just one of those straws you hear about that can so easily can break the camel's back.

Then stabbing unbearable pain in the gut! OMG . . . I can feel the knives stabbing and tearing my gut to pieces. It hurts so much, I am screaming out in pain . . . Why don't I just pass out? Please just let it end, I have to make this all end!

This is when my thoughts become a serious desire. I needed to get my gun. I needed to put an end to this. The word "unbearable" does not, cannot, convey how bad I felt.

What is the point? This is not living.

So here we were – clinical depression. No appetite, bottom of the barrel sadness because it is never going to get better. Needing a break, hoping for a break, but instead having more crap piled on.

The kids didn't know who I was anymore. To them, I was just the ogre that lives by himself at the end of the hall.

Carrie was great, though. In so many ways she worked to keep it all together. Many days when I could not get to the dinner table, Carrie brought dinner and the boys to me. Many evenings she gathered up all three boys and deposited them on the couch, the floor and the bed with us in the bedroom so we could all watch our favorite TV shows together and catch up on the joys and sorrows of daily life.

My wife loves me, but I am afraid that someday she will decide that it is okay to get more out of life than I have been able to give her.

I try. I try harder than she knows, but I only have so much. I will myself every day to be present in her life. Only time will tell if it is enough.

So why am I still here?

Because God gave me my own personal angel. Just as Christopher and my need to raise him allowed me to survive the cancer and all the horrible treatments in the beginning. Carrie is here . . . She is here now to give me the hope and help I need to survive. As long as she is here helping me, counting on me, I cannot let her down. I don't want to let her down, I just can't.

I just can't wait to see what God has in store for us in the future. So I find the strength to hold on for just one more day, and then another. For the first three months of 2010, I just slowly continued a terrifying slide down and farther down into a deep dark depression. Further into the mental and physical darkness I descended.

I don't know why my pain is so horrible . . . That is one of the many frustrating things about all of this. Sometimes I know why I hurt, but other times I have no idea why it is so extreme. Give me cause and effect, I can deal with that. But worse . . . way worse is for no reason; tough for me to deal with that.

I am happy to say that the grip that Carrie has on me did not slip. I am still here and things are much better. I am by no means well, but I am no longer looking for an exit!

So if you ever feel, as I did that there is no reason to go on. That you can no longer take it . . . Wait. Wait at least one more day, see what tomorrow brings. Accept the love and the help of the people in your life.

Had I got my gun (and I was so close), I would have missed soooo much. The only things in life that really matter are our personal relationships. Nurture them, value them, and let them carry you over troubled waters. There is beauty in the trip and on the other shore.

Chapter 31

In Everyone's life, at some time, our inner fire goes out. It is then burst into flame by an encounter with another human being. We should all be thankful for those people who rekindle the spirit.

~ Albert Schweitzer

No Longer a Joke

Many times in my life, I have jokingly said "My get up and go, got up and went!" Well, it finally came true, and it was no longer a joke.

For months, I'd had less and less energy. I could feel ME slipping away a little more all the time; unable to remember the last time I woke up rested and ready to take on the day.

I met with my oncologist and described my concerns; no energy, difficulty thinking clearly, and after my latest increase in morphine, a complete loss of sex drive.

"Oh, hypogonadism. We'll do a blood test to confirm but I'm sure that's what it is," Dr. Pierce said rather quickly. Apparently, hypogonadism is a byproduct of chemotherapy and high doses of opiates (I deal with both). Lucky me!

Hypogonadism can also cause mental and emotional changes. As testosterone decreases, men experience symptoms similar to those of menopause in women. These include: fatigue, decreased sex drive, difficulty concentrating and hot flashes, *"just a case of the vapors darling."*

Dr. Pierce ordered a complete blood workup and started me on AndroGel. It is a topical gel form of testosterone. The kind of thing that muscle builders would love to get their hands on! Most men get shots, but because of my Coumadin use that would not be safe for me, as it thins out my blood to prevent clots.

It turns out that my free testosterone level was about 14½% of the minimum it should be. So once a day, I get to smear a couple tubes of AndroGel on my abdomen and right shoulder. The right shoulder, because Carrie snuggles up on my left side, and my abdomen because Jennifer does not wear gloves during physical therapy, and they were both sure they would not look good with a new mustache. People of the female persuasion, must steer clear of AndroGel, unless they look forward to acquiring many male traits.

Carrie said she was afraid that I might have been faking my desire with her. It took a while to help her understand what was happening, but I finally came up with an analogy.

I have always been a butt man. I explained that normally if I saw an amazing butt my subconscious would say, "Wow, that's hot." And I would feel a pinch or twinge in my loins. That just doesn't happen anymore.

The other part, the part that never went away, is I see my wife and I know how much I love her. I know how sexy she is. And I want to hold her, caress her and make love with her so she knows how I feel.

This is what it came down to, two different kinds of sex: the "I am horny and I want to resolve that with you" and the "I love you, my wife, and I want to make love with you to show you how much."

The second part is still here, but I want the first part back. The mental part is still here; I just want the physical part back too and not just for sex.

How much better will my life be when I have more energy? When I can be productive for more than 12 hours in a week. I am hopeful, but at the same time afraid to get too excited, just in case.

Tick tock . . . only time will tell . . . tick tock

Chapter 32

Let us rise up and be thankful; for if we didn't learn a lot today, at least we learned a little, and if we didn't learn a little, at least we didn't get sick, and if we got sick, at least we didn't die; so, let us all be thankful.

~ Buddha

What Life Looks Like Today

You know that phrase, "What you see is what you get?" Well, from a health standpoint, it's not true for me. If you saw me on the street, in the line at the grocery store, or even if you were watching one of my keynote speeches, what you see is not what I get. What you see is a big man, a strong man, 250 pounds, 6'3" tall, and most the time you will see a smile from ear to ear. The smile is not fake, it's not like I'm unhappy. The alternative to my situation is death. So yeah, I'm smiling because I'm still alive.

Here's the part you don't see. As you learned in my story, the doctors were sure that I would not survive the cancer. Thank goodness they were wrong and I'm still alive. Due to the severity of the surgery and damage to the nerve tree at the base of my spine, the doctors were sure I was going to be paralyzed from the waist down and be in a wheelchair. As you now know, I'm not paralyzed. The doctors told me I was most likely going to end up with a colostomy bag hanging off my waist. Despite their predictions I am very happy to say that failed to happen as well. But, damage was done. Damage you don't see, but that I deal with every day.

My bowels and bladder were left completely incontinent immediately following the surgery. They would let loose at any time without warning. What it means in real life is my system didn't know or care that I was standing in a line at the grocery store. My plumbing didn't know and didn't care that I was on a date with a beautiful woman. My plumbing still doesn't know or care that I'm standing in front of 200 people making a speech. Because of the nerve damage I don't even feel it happening. Unfortunately sometimes people around me know before I do.

So for the first three years I got to wear what was affectionately called an "adult nighttime protection device." For me it wasn't just nighttime, no... I got to wear them 24 hours a day, seven days a week. I think you all know it by a different name, a diaper. Want to take a minute and think about whether or not you would have a smile on your face from ear to ear as you continually and unexpectedly dealt with these problems? Not fun. Very demoralizing, humiliating even.

The bladder and bowel nerves were not the only nerves to be damaged. In addition to incontinence, I got impotence. It was promised, it was not unexpected. So there I was a man who always had a very healthy appetite when it came to female companionship, not able to function. A smile on your face ear-to-ear huh?

I had a choice. I could say that because of these problems life is not worth living. I could have chosen to say that there is nothing to be thankful for. I could have resigned myself to the fact that this is the way life was going to be forever and that I could never be happy with that.

But like I shared with you before, I have succeeded in my life with that simple two-step process; Decide then Do. I decided to be happy, and for the most part, I was. I decided to do everything I could to make the most of my life and I did. I decided to work to get every improvement in every facet of my life that I could, and I have.

With a strong positive mental attitude and a continued fight forward step-by-step, things have improved. There has been some nerve regeneration. What does that mean in day-to-day life? It means I don't have to wear adult night guard protection 24 hours a day seven days a week anymore. The downside is I don't know which days I have to, and which days I don't, until it's too late. But it's getting better, and that's the part I focus on. And the impotence, that's gotten dramatically better. So many things can be improved and controlled and manipulated by our mental powers. In my mind knowing how much my wife loves me, and knowing how beautiful and sexy she is, has allowed me to function as a loving husband.

Is everything perfect, now? No. Sometimes my bowels leak without warning, sometimes my bladder leaks without warning. It frustrates the living hell out of me. But then I stop and think as bad as this is, as bad as this is... would I, for one-minute, trade it for being dead. The answer is always, "No, I'll take this over death."

Pain, now that's a different story. You can't see it. I don't let you. I hide it so well now – still that smile ear to ear. Getting ready to travel requires bed rest so that I can tolerate the pain of sitting in a car or on an airplane for several hours. After I get off the stage, it's two or three days in bed recuperating. The pain is so intense and exhausting that I hope and pray to be able to sleep most of that time away. After a few days, I am able to come out of my "cave" and rejoin my family in day-to-day life. But my day-to-day life is also affected by my pain.

One of the most effective ways for me to deal with my pain is to use biofeedback, positive mental imaging and mind control. I first learned the basics while in high school at Washington Union. I was on the track team participating in several events. The one that gave me the most trouble was the high jump. As long as the bar was below my eye level I could clear it. In fact I could clear it by a wide margin. But once the bar got to my eye level, I would just crash into it. It was obviously a mental problem, with the bar just one inch below eye level I could clear it by almost a foot, but raised up to eye level and . . . crash!

Someone give me a book about mind control. The ideas put forth in that book allowed me to break through the mental barrier I had dealing with that bar. I learned to visualize myself clearing that bar over and over again until it became real and possible. Once that bar and I got to see eye to eye, I could clear it. I realized that I could use the techniques that I learned from that book in all areas of my life.

The main way I deal with pain is by climbing into a beautiful hammock on the beach and in my mind I'm really there. Soft, white rope braided in a perfect pattern. (Carrie says when my pain is bad she can see me rub the rope between my fingers over and over again, even though I'm asleep). Wooden spars hold the hammock open as it swings in the gentle breeze. This amazing hammock is suspended between two very tall palm trees. It sways softly with the gentle breeze coming off the water. Water so blue it is hard to believe that it is real, but it is real because I have been there, and I get to go back whenever I wish. To calm my mind, I focus on a place, a time, and surrounding so beautiful and so peaceful. It allows me to create a new reality and let the pain drift away. I think it is like laughing, it is hard to be mad or feel bad when you are really laughing. I mean losing yourself in an amazing moment, a giant, bending-over belly laugh.

For every physical thing I do, I must pay a huge price in pain. So I ration the time I am up and active carefully; it's only three hours a day on a good day. Many days I'm faced with the difficult decision of whether or not to be productive with my work, or to spend time with my family. Do I write another chapter or take the kids to a movie? Do I work on a project around the house or do I take Carrie out wine tasting? I don't have the luxury of doing both. I can only do one or the other. I want so much to be able to do it all like I used to. It weighs heavily on me, but then I remember my favorite saying… "Every day that I wake up and I'm not dead, well, that's a good day."

What about the cancer you ask? Let me tell you as time passed and more and more tests came back negative for new cancer Dr. Pierce's demeanor lightened up becoming more and more jovial with each new visit. Then recently he came into the exam room with a smile on his face saying, "Davido, Davido! How are you doing Davido?" This was the first time he ever called me that. "Davido, I think you have beaten this… you are a very lucky man!"

Chapter 33

True enough, we all have obligations and duties toward our fellow men. But it does seem curious enough that in modern, neurotic society, men's energies are consumed in making a living, and rarely in living itself. It takes a lot of courage for man to declare, with clarity and simplicity, that the purpose of life is to enjoy it.

~ the pleasures of a nonconformist

(I have carried a copy of this quote in my wallet for most of my adult life.)

Always Remember…

Everyone has the capacity to change his or her life. No one else is going to do it for you. All of my life I have followed a very simple and straightforward approach.

"Decide . . . Then do!" Yes, it is that easy.

Most people just never get off the dime because they are afraid they will fail. Maybe you will, maybe you won't. But I can guarantee that never trying ensures the very failure that you are afraid of.

Not succeeding every time you try something is not failing, it just moves you one step closer to getting what you want. We have all heard the stories of Thomas Edison and his quest for the light bulb. Each time it did not work, he learned something new that moved him one step closer to success.

I have always thought of it as a beautiful sailboat, sleek lines, a gorgeous yacht. While she is at anchor nothing changes, nothing gets better. Then you raise your anchor and the sails and set out for your destination, what you picture in your mind is your success. Off you set sail, maybe you don't see the progress that you hoped for. What do you do? You adjust your course and move ever closer to your destination! Remember it doesn't always work out as a straight course; Edison made thousands of course adjustments, never quitting and finally reaching success. You can too – just don't give up.

The point is, while you sit at anchor not moving, you will never achieve your goals. Tilt your head back, close your eyes, let the sun warm your face; let the breeze blow through your hair. Raise your sails and set off on your adventure, because while you're at anchor nothing changes, but by simply setting sail you can adjust your course and reach your goals!

So here we are at the end of our journey together, as I write this

I am waiting, not very patiently I might add, for yet another test. Yes by the time you read this we will all know the results, but I have to stop somewhere. My story goes on, new chapters to write, new adventures to relish. Even after I die, my story goes on, not just in this book but also in the people I love. Christopher who has had a lifetime of lessons from me. Carrie who I know I have touched but not as much as she has touched me. Garret and Mitchel, I can only hope that the short time I have gotten with them leaves them with warmth in their heart and a few tools to make life a little easier and more understandable.

I lay here in bed typing away, wondering if you did indeed enjoy the ride. Gosh I hope so. Will you use some of the hard lessons I shared to improve your life? Will you pick up the phone and call that person you know you need to call, just tell them that you love them no matter what – the rest is just small stuff. You know what they say, don't sweat the small stuff. Will you get out of your chair and walk into the family room and give your partner a great big hug . . . Just hold them for what seems the longest time, then give them a kiss, the way you would like to be kissed?

Find your dad or your mom, find your son or your daughter, and tell them how you feel, no codes, no secrets just tell them. Tell all of the people in your life what you would say as if you knew you would be gone tomorrow. Because we just never know when our time is up and love like that should be shared and nurtured, allowed to grow, and to nourish each of you.

You can check in on me and my family by going to my website:

www.somedaygroup.com

I will be traveling around doing readings and signing books. Carrie and I will be appearing all over this great planet of ours, sharing our stories and working to help those who come to listen. We have learned many of life's lessons the hard way and, if you will do us the honor, we would love to help you avoid the potholes we have found and benefit from the lessons we learned being so close to death.

Until we meet, thank you! And please live your life to the fullest. Always remembering that...

"Today is someday!"

My Creed

I do not choose to be a common man. It is my right to be uncommon… if I can.

I seek opportunity… not security. I do not wish to be a kept citizen, humbled and dulled by having the state look after me. I want to take the calculated risk; to dream and to build, to fail and to succeed.

I refuse to barter incentive for a dole. I prefer the challenges of life to the guaranteed existence; the thrill of fulfillment to the stale calm of utopia.

I will not trade freedom for beneficence nor my dignity for a handout. I will never cower before any master nor bend to any threat. It is my heritage to stand erect, proud and unafraid; to think and act for myself; enjoy the benefits of my creations and to face the world boldly and say, this I have done

All this is what it means to be an American.

~ Dean Alfange

CPSIA information can be obtained at www.ICGtesting.com
Printed in the USA
BVOW071446161211

278550BV00001B/13/P

9 781432 774486